EAT HEALTHY,
BE HEALTHY –
IT IS THAT SIMPLE!

LIZ GRAYBILL

Eat Healthy, Be Healthy - It is that Simple!

ISBN: 10: 1978187939
ISBN-13: 978-1978187931

To my family and my extended family,
"I love you all so much. Please eat healthy to
be healthy."

Contents

ACKNOWLEDGMENTS

God placed on my heart to write this book and share my knowledge on healthy eating. Thanks be to God!

Also, to my wonderful and loving husband, Doug Graybill. None of this book would have been written if it was not for you encouraging me and holding me accountable. You graciously allowed me the time I needed to accomplish writing my book. Never once did you complain when I said I was enrolling in an online course to learn about health and nutrition or to learn to write a book. If fact, you always said "You better go do your course." Thank you so much for your love and support! I love you so much.

To my sister-in-law, Michaele Christiansen, thank you so much for allowing me to walk with you every night for 50 minutes. I really needed those hills! I walk faster and further with you than I walk on my own. My toned legs are due to the hilly course you selected for our fast-paced walks. Thank you.

I had a few other encouragers along the way that I would like to acknowledge.

Carol Mikosz and Mike Mescavage who both were behind the scene encouraging me to write a book to share my knowledge on health. Those two often stated how they thought my daily healthy Facebook tips were very helpful and informative. Your encouragement helped me more than you will ever know! Thank you so much Carol and Mike. Also, thank you to all my faithful Facebook followers who took the time to read, "like" and or comment on my daily healthy tips.

I would be remiss if I did not mention my short-legged Jack Russell terrier, Max. When I did not want to walk, Max always needed to walk. When I wanted to walk, Max wanted to run. When I had no energy to walk, Max had energy. He was always ready to walk, rain or shine. Thanks Max, you helped me so much. Love you little walking buddy!

INTRODUCTION

The most important thing you can do for your health is to eat healthy. Many people overlook the fact that eating healthy will heal you. Eating unhealthy foods will make you sick, full of ailments, diseases and literally make you unhealthy. Usually turning to one's diet is the last thing so many of us do and it should be the first thing we do. It is simple to eat healthy, we just have to learn what eating healthy is and then do it. Eat healthy for life not as a short-term diet.

I was going to specifically title one chapter "It Worked for Me!" but if you are anything like me, as you are standing in the book store and you come across a chapter titled "It Worked for Me!" you are going to open to that chapter and start reading it standing right there. Everyone wants to know what works so they too can get results. Read this book from cover-to-cover and then you will see first-hand and understand what worked for me.

I am going to share my story of eating unhealthily, being overweight, tired all the time, no energy, and having thyroid issues. I will share with you how I learned to eat healthier, have more energy, and how eating healthy cleared my thyroid issues. I will teach you how simple it is to eat healthy. Eating healthy was the reason I lost 30 pounds. I did not take diet pills, drink meal replacement shakes, take weight loss sticks, nothing like that. I lost my weight by learning to eat healthy. I went from being overweight to now being a Certified Health Coach. I went from not knowing what foods were healthy to now eating healthier every day. I cannot emphasize enough how important it is for your health that you eat healthy!

It is simple to eat healthy. I will share with you many simple ways to improve your eating habits so you too will be eating your way to better health. Eating healthy is not a diet rather it is a way of life.

What does eating healthy mean to you? Take a moment now to visualize what eating healthy means for you. Everyone has their own definition of what eating healthy means to them. I asked one person what eating healthy meant to them and they said eating more plant based foods and more fish. To me, eating healthy means several things like eating better cleaner foods, eating more whole foods and plant based foods, eating less meats, eating less processed foods, eating foods with fewer ingredients, making better and healthier choices, and I could go on and on as to what eating healthy means to me.

As a Certified Health Coach, I help people who are ready: ready to want to learn to eat healthier and who are ready to lose weight. As a Health Coach, I ask a lot of questions to my clients and listen to their answers so I can better help them on their healthy journey. In this book, I write as if I am sitting there talking to you, so I ask a lot of questions. I help people to reach their goals and help to bring balance into all areas of their life. I teach them healthier food options thus helping them improve their diets so they can be eating healthier to be healthy. Eating and being healthy involves more than the foods we choose to put on our plates. Stress, work, relationships, emotions and so much more affects what we eat and therefore affects our health.

In this self-help book, I will mainly focus on eating healthy but other topics have an impact on our health and will be discussed. I do not lay out step-by-step or number the steps you should take to be healthy. As you read the book you will notice all my ideas, what worked for me, my mistakes and you can translate all of these into a step-by-step guide. As you read my story of becoming healthier, my goal is that you let it inspire you and transform you as I was transformed.

I will share some mantras that helped me stay focused on my goals. The information in this book will help people to eat better and to be on their way to being healthier. Understand that we are all different, we all have different goals, we all have different tastes, and different illnesses. This book is written with basic steps to teach everyone how simple it is to eat healthier and how simple it is to make better food choices. Truly the hardest step for many of us is to just start, whether it is starting to eat healthy or starting a daily routine, starting is the hardest step.

I suggest you read this self-help book cover-to-cover the first time through. You will learn what helped me to become healthier and lose weight. After reading through the book once, you may want to use it as a guide to keep you motivated and moving forward on your healthy journey.

I recommend you get a notebook or a journal and use it along with reading this book. When I ask a question, really think about the answer, then put your answer in your notebook or journal. Do not just read the question and keep reading. Take time to think about the question being asked and jot down your answer to the question in your notebook or journal. In the "Let's Get Started" chapter, there are blank lines for you to put your answer to some questions. I recommend you put those answers here in the book and also in your notebook or journal. The more thought you put into the question and your answers, the more you will be transformed. If you put in the work, you will see results. If you are just reading the words and not working through the steps, you will have a harder time getting the results you dream of.

My goal for each of you is that the next time you go to your doctor, your doctor says "I'm not sure what you are doing, but your numbers look great. Whatever you are doing, keep doing it!" A doctor telling you that you are healthy is one my definitions of being healthy.

Are you ready to begin your journey to being healthy by taking simple steps to improve the foods you are eating? Get ready to be transformed! Are you ready to hear my story?

Chapter 1

My Personal Story: Overweight to being a Certified Health Coach

I grew up as a very fussy eater. I ate the same foods every day for many years. My family ate everything and because I was a fussy eater, I only ate a few foods, over and over, day in and day out. I grew up eating hot creamy chocolate cereal every morning for breakfast. Growing up, I ate a lot of processed boxed macaroni and cheese and canned tomato soup. My mother would always prepare me the foods that I ate, basically preparing two separate meals, mine and theirs. When I was in 8th grade, my mother was in the hospital for a while so my father became the cook. He made me try everything that he cooked. I gained twenty pounds that year! I learned to like hamburgers, pizza, mashed potatoes and many more foods.

I went into the U.S. Army when I was almost 19 years old. In basic training, our food was served to us. You ate what they put on your plate. In basic training, I was scared to death of my drill sergeants. When they said to eat everything on my plate, I did exactly that. In basic training is when I started eating vegetables, and only because they were on my plate. The drill sergeants would say "you have ten minutes to eat and nine minutes are already gone!" I learned to eat fast, basically "eat now and taste it later" concept. I was stationed everywhere while in the military including stationed in different countries. I had the opportunity to experience many different cultures as well as their foods. I then learned to eat and like a lot of different foods. I was now eating many different foods and I gained weight. After only 5 years in the military, I became overweight and I was no longer a fussy eater. I was overweight by military standards. I was not proud of the fact that I was now overweight. I had to be taped, which means I had to be measured every six months. Literally, they would measure my neck, wrist, forearm, and hips with a tape measure. Then a formula was used to see exactly how much bodyfat I had. I always carried my weight well and did not appear overweight while wearing the uniform. I could perform well on my physical fitness test which consisted of two minutes of push-ups, two minutes of sit-ups and a two-mile run. I would always max my physical fitness test, scoring 100% in each event.   Because I was "overweight" it did not make me feel fit as a Soldier should be even though I was fit. Being overweight and having to be taped all the time did not help with my confidence or my self-esteem. I was in the U.S. Army for 23 years and I was overweight for the last 18 years. That is 18 years of being taped every six months and being told I was overweight. With me being over my recommended body fat each and every tape for 18 years, that was not good for my self-esteem. I thought with all the long-distance runs, the long road marches and everything else physical that we had to do in the military, that I would not have had any weight issue. I am sure you too would have thought just because I was a Soldier and all the physical fitness that we are required to do, that I was to weight standards. But I was not, I was overweight and kept gaining weight. I did not feel good about myself. I often thought to myself, I work out every day, how could I be overweight?   I would even work out each morning on my own for about 30 minutes before Army physical fitness training, which was another hour of working out. I was still overweight!

I was eating everything I wanted, as much as I wanted and expecting to work it off with all the exercise I did in the military. I did not lose weight rather just the opposite, I kept gaining weight. No matter what exercise I did or how much I exercised, I could not lose weight. I started running slower due to my weight. I had no energy to run. I was tired all the time. I was eating poorly and I had no energy, bad combination!

I was overweight, tired all the time, just had no energy and then I was diagnosed with hypothyroidism. As if being overweight, tired, and no energy was not enough. Hypothyroidism meant my thyroid was underactive and not producing enough thyroid hormone. With an underactive thyroid, it caused my body's process to slow down making it harder to lose weight. Therefore, I gained weight and could not lose the weight. I was tired all the time. I constantly had a sluggish feeling, like I just had no energy. Constipation is a side effect of having thyroid issues. I doctored with thyroid issues for about 7 years. The doctors were always changing my thyroid medication because I was all over the charts with my thyroid numbers. Every time my numbers changed, my doctor would adjust my thyroid medicine. Of course, when my medicine was changed, my numbers would change. My numbers were up, down, and all over the charts. It is harder to lose weight when your thyroid is not working as it should be and I just kept gaining weight.

When I would eat out, which was quite often, I felt I always had to order dessert. I felt I had to order dessert even if I was already full. I felt like I was "treating" or "rewarding" myself because I was eating out, like eating out made me authorized to eat dessert. I really thought I could order dessert, especially if I did not eat all my food that I ordered. I looked to dessert after a meal as if I was "treating" myself to something nice. Of course, eating out often, making poor food choices while eating out and ordering dessert were the worst things for my weight. My weight just kept increasing. Yet somehow eating out and ordering dessert all the time made me "think" I felt better. How silly was that, eating out, eating dessert, gaining weight and yet somehow it was supposed to make me feel better about myself. That does not even pass what I call the common-sense test. It does not even make sense when you read it let alone when I was doing it and living it.

If at ate at a restaurant with a salad bar, I thought I was doing myself a favor to eat a lot of the different "salads" on the salad bar.   I would eat coleslaw, ambrosia salad, macaroni salad, and potato salad from salad bars. I never actually ate a green leafy salad with all the fresh vegetables. If I did eat a green leafy salad, I would drench my salad with a lot of the store-bought ranch dressing. If I just choose to eat a lot of the fresh vegetables on the salad bar, I still would drench my vegetables with the salad dressing. Notice I did not say I would dip my vegetables into the salad dressing but would drench my vegetables with the salad dressing. I was eating all the wrong salads at the salad bar yet thinking I was eating a healthy salad. I just did not know how to eat healthy.

I thought eating out was quick, easy and healthy. I never once thought that restaurants would serve food that is unhealthy. I learned it actually takes more time to select a restaurant, drive there, select a meal, eat the meal and come home than it does it prepare and cook a meal at home. So, eating out is not always quicker and if it is, then you are probably eating fast food and that is definitely not healthy foods to be eating. I know restaurants serve large portions, larger than what anyone should be eating at one meal. I never really thought that maybe the food restaurants serve are not the healthiest foods. I trusted restaurants thinking that they had my health in mind when they prepared meals. I learned that is not the case at all! Restaurants want you to like the food they serve so you will keep coming back and back. Just because restaurants serve food, does not mean it is healthy food. When I eat out now, I often think of the price of the meal. If I am paying only a few dollars for a burger than I know I am probably not receiving organic, hormone free, pasture raised beef for the price I am paying for that burger. That thought alone almost makes me sick and not want to eat my burger. When eating out, you cannot control whether you receive organic foods or GMO foods, or even foods pumped full of antibiotics. It is always much healthier to eat at home. When eating at home, you know what foods you have purchased and the quality of that food. Eating out is usually not the healthiest option for anyone to select.

After retiring from the military, I hit my all-time highest weight. I gained about 10 pounds after retiring, and I was already overweight while in the military. Prior to being overweight in the military, I was a size 5 and when I was at my heaviest I was a size 14 maybe even a size 16. I felt awful! I had no energy, I was tired all the time, and I was overweight. I am sure I was quite the sight, a short petite frame woman and overweight.

So, what did I do? I probably did what many of you would do, I spent a couple hundred dollars on tight fitting control top pantyhose, spandex girdles, and tummy slimming body shapers to hold in and hide my fat. I was tired of being overweight and I wanted immediate results. I wanted to be thinner or at least "appear" thinner. Does any of this sound familiar? I never even thought to change the way I was eating. I never thought what I was eating was even causing me to gain weight. How silly of me to think that! I was in denial that "I" could be to blame for my weight. I never even thought that my poor food choices led me to being overweight, how could it right, I was exercising all the time!

Veterans Day was coming up and I needed to fit in my Class A Army uniform for an event. A few days prior to Veterans Day, I bought all those slimming clothes to wear so I could literally "squeeze" into my uniform for the night. Funny thing, I wore all those at the same time, the tight-fitting pantyhose, girdle and tummy slimming body shaper under my military uniform. Want to hear something even funnier? I looked sharp in my uniform that night but I could not sit down and I had to basically take off each layer to go the bathroom! I spent a couple hundred dollars to basically "hide my fat" and not get rid of my fat. How silly was that? That was marketing at its best, advertising control top, spandex, buy larger sizes of clothing instead of advertising to eat healthier to lose the weight. This was my "aha" moment, my turning point to want to lose weight, be healthier and not hide the weight but to lose the weight. I actually was serious this time about losing the weight. I wanted change. I did not want to have to wear tight fitting clothing to hide my fat any longer, rather I wanted to lose the fat for good. I did not just want to appear thinner but I wanted to be thinner.

I thought to myself "what happened to me?" "How did I let myself get so out of shape and so overweight?" I was really not happy with myself, not at all. It was silly of me to think I could eat whatever I wanted, and just exercise it off. It took me a long time to realize it does not work that way!

I then realized it would have been easier to eat healthier to lose the weight so I could fit into my Class A Army uniform than to merely "hide my fat" for one night. I started on my journey to eat healthier and to lose weight.

I did not know where to start nor did I know how to eat healthy. I did not even know portion sizes. I just knew I had to start somewhere. I had to make changes to what I was currently doing since obviously my way was not working. I knew nothing about eating healthy even though I thought I did. My entire adult life, I subscribed to recipe magazines, eating healthy magazines and exercise magazines so I thought I knew how to eat healthy. I never really dieted in my life. I would just try to eat more salads when I knew I would have a military weigh-in coming up but I never really dieted. When I reached my all-time highest weight, I did join a weight loss group for a while. At the time, it was more focused on the number on the scale and not really about eating healthy. I then began drinking detox teas before a weigh-in so I would lose some weight. I even began purging so I would weigh less. I knew these were not the healthiest ways to lose weight. I did not want to continue to do these things to lose weight. I began my journey to healthier eating to feel better and to lose weight by making healthier food choices.

I realized that subscribing to eating healthy magazines and actually reading healthy magazines were two different things. I started getting rid of my old recipe books that were unhealthy. I had a lot of dessert recipe books. They were first to go so I would not be tempted to make desserts. I started making recipes from my healthy magazines. I started noticing portion sizes in photos of recipes. I started eating more salads with more leafy greens and vegetables. I cut out salad dressings. I stopped ordering desserts when I ate out. I started reading the menus to select what I thought was the healthiest meal to order instead of just ordering what sounded good or what looked good. I started reading labels and looking for less ingredients. I started to prepare more foods from scratch using whole foods and actually cooking. I stopped ordering all those fancy coffee drinks that were more like milkshakes than coffee.

It was not until a couple years ago that I learned you cannot exercise your way out of a bad diet. I did not know that! Why wasn't I told that while I was in the Army that you cannot exercise your way out of a bad diet? This was another "aha" moment for me because I did not know you could not eat everything you wanted and expect to work it off. Many people are just like I used to be, thinking they can eat anything and everything, eat as much as they want and just work it off. It does not work that way! You have to change what you eat to lose weight and be healthy and then you can add in exercise, not the other way around. Eat healthy to be healthy, it is that simple!

On my journey to eating healthier, I have lost 30 pounds! The best part is, I have kept off the weight and toned up. I no longer have thyroid issues therefore I no longer take thyroid medication. I am not tired all the time since I no longer have thyroid issues. I have more energy. I eat better and healthier every day. I have clear glowing skin. I'm happier and I feel great! I am comfortable in my own skin and body. I like vegetables now and I am not just eating them because my drill sergeant is telling me to eat them. I enjoy and look forward to exercise and have energy to exercise. I am now in a size 8 or size 9. I do not have to purchase and wear all the tummy slimming spandex body shaping clothing! Nor do I want to wear those types of clothing again.

I have never regretted getting healthier and losing weight! When I got serious about eating healthy, I realized how simple it is to eat healthy. I have learned so much on my own healthy journey and now I want to help others to become healthier. I want to teach others to eat healthy and let them know they do not need to rely on shakes, drinks, meal supplements, meal replacements or diet sticks to lose weight but that they can do it by eating healthy foods.

My healthy journey lead me to becoming a Certified Health Coach. As a Certified Health Coach, I now teach people about eating healthier, eating whole foods, less processed foods and discuss healthier food swaps, food combining, all while trying to bring balance into their life. With my clients, I discuss more than what is covered here in this book, because everyone is unique and has a different path which they want to take.   I help people reach their health goals, not my health goals, but their health goals. I teach them everything I learned on my journey to becoming healthier so they too can become their healthiest self. I share my story to inspire others to eat healthier and to heal their health issues. Food really is everything! Becoming healthier really starts with the foods we eat.

It is never too late to start eating healthy. It is never too late to make your health a priority. There is no such thing as too old or too sick to start eating healthy.

Who would have ever thought that as a fussy eater growing up that I would one day be overweight? Who would have ever thought that I, once overweight, would now be a Certified Health Coach who is teaching others about foods and eating healthy? Your health journey may not lead you to wanting to be a health coach and that is okay. Remember it is your health journey, not mine, that you are striving to achieve. My goals are not your goals.

Eating healthy is the most important thing you can do for your health. There are other little things you can do to improve your overall well-being and health, but eating healthy is the best way. Are you ready to learn about eating healthy and other little things to do to improve your health? Great, let's get started!

Chapter 2

Let's Get Started

Do you find it hard to just start? Do you wonder where to start and how to get started? You will not have to wonder any longer how to get started, I am going to help you! In this chapter, I am going to give you several simple ideas or rather simple steps to help you get started. These ideas are simple steps that you can implement into your daily life that will help you to start and then maintain your healthy journey. I wanted to write this entire book and start each paragraph with "Start" because starting is the hard part. But once you start, you are well on your way to doing and maintaining what you started. Look at your new healthy journey as many "starts." You are starting a new way of eating. You are starting a healthier lifestyle. You are starting to make yourself a priority and take care of yourself in ways that you never have before. You can select all of these simple ideas to help you get started or you can select the ones that you know you will use. Maybe you will want to try a few ideas mentioned here then add in more ideas from this chapter at a later time.

I am sure you heard it said before to "just start and do it for five minutes." That could apply to pretty much anything in life. Just start reading your Bible five minutes a day. Just start with an exercise you like and do it for five minutes. Just start cleaning out your closet and do it for five minutes. The idea behind saying a time limit is for the hope that you will get into it and keep going, not even thinking about the five minutes you told yourself you would do. If you start to read your Bible for five minutes a day, will you really stop reading when five minutes are up even if you are in the middle of reading a sentence or in the middle of reading a chapter? Same goes with "just starting" anything, are you going to stop after five minutes of walking around the block or are you going to continue walking around the block until you complete the block? I am asking you to just start eating healthier, and you will see how simple it really is. Just start and see for yourself how simple it is to eat healthy. Just start, you will not regret it.

It is so important that you learn to eat healthy if you want to be healthy. Many people do not even realize that the foods they eat can make them healthy or unhealthy. I know I did not realize that! Food is the number one thing making us overweight, obese, and sick. The list of ailments and diseases goes on and on. Who knew that food could turn a disease around? Food is also the number one thing that can make us healthy. Amazing! Who would have ever thought that food can do all that. Food really is everything. I cannot emphasize enough how important it is for you to eat healthy so that you will be healthy, it is that simple! Often times people make changes to their diet, to the food they eat as a last resort and not the first resort. When in reality, what a person eats should be the first thing that is looked at as causing their illnesses.

No matter where you are at in your life, young or old, unhealthy or wanting to be healthier, it is so important that you just start where you are at. Just start! Start with the basics and build on them as you learn more. You do not have to be perfect to start but you do have to start before you will see results. I think part of that sentence is powerful and needs to be repeated so you get the gist of it: you do have to "start," take action, before you will see results. You do not have to know everything there is to know about eating healthy before you start, you just have to start somewhere with your eating. Start one day, you pick the day and start first thing in the morning. Start with one day, one meal to add in at least one healthy food. Start with one meal a week and begin making it to be a healthier meal.

First you have to have a goal. If you do not have a goal, you surely will not reach it. Without a goal, you will be doing anything and everything with no real goal in sight. You will not be accomplishing anything because you will not know what you are striving to reach. What is your goal? Your goal will be different than my goal. You may even have several goals and that is fine.

When I started on my journey to eating healthier a couple years ago, my goal was to lose weight, period. I just wanted to lose weight. What is your goal? Is your goal to lose weight? Maybe your goal is to gain weight (not everyone wants to lose weight)?

Is your goal to get healthy? Is your goal to eat foods with five ingredients or less? Is your goal to eat less processed foods? Is your goal to cut out added sugars? Is your goal to lose belly fat? Do you want to eat healthy to have more energy? Maybe your goal is to run a 5k race some day? Maybe your goal is to go off a couple of your medications? Whatever your goal is, you have to have a goal. Your goal may be different than my starting goal and that is okay.

Please take a few moments now to list your top three health goals. (Remember to also list your top three health goals in your new healthy journal or healthy notebook that you will be using along with reading this book.)

1. _______________________________
2. _______________________________
3. _______________________________

Then I needed to know "why" I wanted to lose weight. I had to have a "why", something that would keep me moving toward my goal to lose weight. My "why" I wanted to lose weight was to be able to breathe. I say that because I felt as if every meal I ate was more like a Thanksgiving meal. I was always so full after I ate that it made me feel as though I could not breathe. I guess my stomach was so full it would push on my diaphragm and it made it difficult for me to breathe. I do have allergies to many different things and asthma so it does make it hard to breathe at times. It was scary at times when I felt I could not breath properly, especially if I ate in the evening and then went to bed with a very full stomach, I just could not breathe normally. I knew I had to lose weight because I did not like that constant full stomach feeling and the feeling of not being able to breathe. My other "why" was to be able to fit into my Class A Army uniform.

Now you have to have a "why?" Why are these your top three health goals? Why do you want to get healthy? What would "healthy" look like for you? What are the benefits for you to reach your health goals? Your "why" has to be so strong that it will make you want to get out of bed every day and take action so you will reach your goal.

What is your "why'? Please think about your "why" and write your "why" remembering to make it so strong that it will drive you to reach your goal.

Your "why" you want to be healthy:

____

____

____

Writing down your goal and your "why" and keeping them visible will help you to stay focused on reaching your goal.   A journal or even a 3x5 index card will be sufficient. Writing your goal and your "why" is like a contract with yourself. It makes it more real when it is written instead of just thinking it. It is also a daily visual for you to reach your goal. Remember, it is your goal, not my goal for you, it is your goal.

Have you ever heard of a SMART goal? SMART stands for specific, measurable, achievable, realistic and timed goal. Sometimes we set a goal for ourselves and it is not a specific enough goal. Maybe it is not even a realistic goal or it is a goal without a date to reach the goal. When I said "I want to lose weight" that is not a SMART goal. I was not specific in the amount of weight I wanted to lose. It was measurable because I could weigh myself to see if I lost weight or I could use my clothes as a better indicator to see if I was losing weight. I could even use my overall health as an indicator to how I felt. I did not even say I wanted to lose weight by a specific date, like for an upcoming wedding or for an upcoming vacation. There was no time line for me to reach my goal. My goal was not a SMART goal. How many times have you set a goal for yourself and it was not even a realistic goal, or a SMART goal? The chances of reaching your goal when it is not a SMART goal or a realistic goal are very slim (no pun intended).

It was a September day when I set my SMART goal to lose weight by Veterans Day. I started in September which was smart in itself because it allowed me time to reach my goal of losing weight to fit into my Class A Army uniform. Usually I would just get serious that I needed to lose weight a few days prior to Veterans Day each year so I could fit into my uniform, and by that time, it was always too late to sensibly lose the weight. But this time was different, I wanted it to be specific, realistic and lose the weight healthily by Veterans Day.

Take your top three goals that you wrote above and re-write them to make each goal a SMART goal.

1._______________________

____

____

____

____

____

2._______________________

____

____

____

3._______________________

____

____

____

____

____

Now you have to set mini goals which will help you reach your SMART goal. I like to call this little action steps that you will take to reach your bigger goal. I do this using reverse planning. You know your goal and when you want to reach your goal and now you have to do reverse planning which are the mini steps you will take to get to your goal. Your goal is probably a long-term goal so you need short-term goals or mini goals to get you to your long-term goal. These mini goals will be in line with your goal. If your long-term goal is to lose 50 pounds in 1 year, then your mini goal may be to lose 1 to 2 pounds per week, each week for a year to reach your goal. The reverse planning then would be to say what do I need to do each week to be losing 1 to 2 pounds to reach my long-term goal. You will need to be tweaking, altering, modifying and changing your food intake and may need to increase your exercise to reach your goal of losing 1 to 2 pounds a week. For mini goals, you are stating for each week or each day you will commit to doing specific things to keep you on track and in line with your goal. Look at it as action steps that you can take that will constantly be bringing you closer to your goal.

What are a few of your mini goals that will help you stay on track to reach your goal?

1. ___________________________________

____

2. ___________________________________

____

3. ______________________________

____

Another great place to help you get started is to take a photo of yourself. A photo is a great place to begin. Let this be the "before" photo because you will be losing weight and transforming and you will never look like this again. This photo will be a great visual to keep you on track. With a photo, you will be able to see results and this will keep you moving forward. Periodically, keep taking updated photos of yourself. You will see your clothes fitting loser and maybe you will see your skin getting more vibrant looking and you will see yourself overall getting healthier. When you take a photo of yourself, please do not beat yourself up over how you look or how you let yourself get like that. The photo is a "before" photo **only** and not for you to critique yourself negatively.

A journal is another great place to start. A journal lets you see exactly what you are eating, how much you are eating, your feelings around eating and so much more. You can journal if you ate because it was breakfast, lunch or dinner or did you eat because you were hungry, angry, or stressed. There are many different journals out there to select from or you can just use a notebook. Select a journal that you like and will use. Make it "feel" good to use the journal. If the journal does not fit your needs, maybe it is asking too many questions or having you track things you do not want to track, consider buying and using a different journal. A journal is a great visual to show you exactly how much food you ate on any given day and what type of foods you ate. It also will be great to show your progress with the changes in your food as you begin eating healthier. After tracking in a journal, you will see where you may want to make modifications or changes in your diet and eating habits.

A Gratitude Journal is another great idea. As you are making progress and putting it in your Gratitude Journal it keeps you focused on the positives and not the negatives in your life. Get in the habit each day before bed to lists three things you are grateful for and you cannot ever list the same things again. Each day three new things you are grateful for so that means you have to read back a couple days ensuring you do not list the same thing again. Gratitude brings more gratitude and that attracts more positive things in your life. Want to be happy? Then start a Gratitude

Journal and you will be surprised how quickly you start noticing the positives in your life and not the negatives. Being grateful helps you to be overall healthier.

Scheduling everything really does help you to get started and to remain on track with your healthy journey. Schedule everything, schedule and plan your menu, grocery shopping, and meal preparation. Schedule time to work out. Schedule time for yourself. I even schedule time to clean my house. On specific days and specific times, I clean a certain part of my house. Scheduling helps things that need to be done and are important to you to be done repetitiously, and become second nature. Now scheduling is second nature to me. I know every Monday morning I am washing my bedding, cleaning ceiling fans, and cleaning air conditioner filters.   If time allows then I will vacuum and mop on Mondays, if not then that will be done on Tuesday. When you block time for your health, then you are making you and your health a priority. Until you make yourself a priority, you will never make time for your health. You are important, I want you to know that and I want you to believe it. You are important so make time for you and your health. Start scheduling everything on your calendar or cell phone calendar that is important to you. Then do what you have on your calendar scheduled to do. Follow through with what you say you will do.

Are you ready to start? I mean are you really ready to start? Is your attitude ready? If you are not ready, no matter what I say and what advice I give, if you are not ready, you will not implement anything I am saying. You have to be open-minded to trying new foods and switching things up. If you will not try new things, are you really ready to eat healthier to get healthier?

As you are getting started, do not think of it as giving up your favorite foods or restricting calories. Rather think of it as new opportunities to in add in new and healthier foods. It is simple, fun and interesting to experiment and try new foods. You may even find new recipes that you like even better than the foods you are currently eating. Take a vegetable that you know you like and prepare it differently. If you are used to eating that vegetable raw now try steaming it or boiling it. Maybe you usually slice a vegetable so now try dicing it as it may taste different to you. Instead of opening a can of vegetables, try buying the same vegetable fresh and noticing the texture and flavor will be so much better. Canned and frozen foods are good but you cannot go wrong with buying fresh.

Remember, if you always do what you have always done, you will always get the same results. The choice is yours to make, do you want to remain the same or do you want to make changes? Do you want to give eating healthy a try to see if your health will improve or not? It is that simple decision to eat healthy that just may transform you and your life for the better. Again, I say the choice is yours alone to make. Do you want different results? Then you have to do things differently. It is that simple.

You may be thinking you have to buy a lot of food before you get started. Or you may be thinking you have to purchase a lot of exercise clothing before you start. You are either ready or you are not ready, those are your only choices. No more procrastination. No more excuses! Maybe you are a little hesitant to get started, maybe you had bad experiences with diets or trying to lose weight in the past. This time will be different, I am going to help you and show you exactly how simple it is to get started and then help you along the way with more ideas and recommendations. That is what a Health Coach does, keep you accountable so you will reach your goal. Just start! You can do it!

I know it is hard to take the first step. I know the hardest part is to just start. Change is scary for everyone. Sometimes we find it easier to stay in our comfort zone even if it means being sick, making poor choices, and being unhealthy. I believe starting has to do more with your mental attitude than your physical ability. You have to be mentally ready to start. You have to want to start and want to be transformed. Start small, start with baby steps.   Just start and you will be on the path to better health.

In the military, we learn by the crawl, walk, run method. Baby steps to start, just learn to crawl and then you will be walking soon enough. As you learn what eating healthy is and you do it consistently for a while, you are then in the walking phase. You will then be able to tweak your diet more and you will be well on your way to better eating and better health. That is the running phase when you know what you are doing, doing it daily and perfecting it for you.

Today, just start drinking half your body weight in ounces of water. If you weigh 200 pounds, then you would drink 100 ounces of water a day. If you weigh 100 pounds then you would drink 50 ounces of water a day. It is actually easy to drink your recommended water a day. When you wake up, since you just went all night without drinking anything, drink one to two cups of water so you get hydrated. Drink a cup of water about 30 minutes before you eat breakfast. Drink a cup of water mid-morning. Drink a cup of water about 30 minutes before eating lunch and dinner. Drink a cup of water mid-afternoon. Drink another cup of water before you go to bed. (You are probably doing the math and thinking that does not add up to even 100 ounces, but you get the idea. You can drink more or less, just be sipping water throughout the day.) You will need to drink more water if you are sweating, exercising or outside on hot humid days. If you are thirsty, you should have already drunk water before you are thirsty. Drink does not mean guzzle but sip your water and enjoy it. You may want to drink more than one cup before meals. Be sipping water all day long. When you are hydrated you will feel better, have more energy, your skin will look better, and you will feel fuller. When you are drinking enough water, you will not have room for sodas, or all those sugary drinks. If you want to drink less coffee, staying hydrated with water is a great place to start because you will not have room for coffee when you are drinking enough water. If you drink caffeinated beverages or alcohol drinks, then you will want to drink one cup of water then your caffeinated beverage or alcohol drink (a one-to-one ratio with drinking the water first).   Water helps to flush out your toxins from your body too. If you find water boring, you can add a few slices of cucumber to your water or watermelon pieces to flavor your water. Distilled water is the best water to be drinking but drink whatever water you have, just be drinking your recommended water each day.

Eat healthy, be healthy - it is that simple! Get back to the basics and start there. When you are eating healthier, it is best to eat whole foods or as close to their natural state as possible. Eating foods with more than five ingredients is when you start getting more into processed foods which means more chemicals and ingredients in your food. You do not have to be a vegetarian or a vegan to be healthy. You will however want to start looking for ways to incorporate eating more whole foods and more plant-based foods into your meals. Think very basic when selecting healthier foods. It is better to eat an orange than to drink store bought orange juice as an orange is in its natural state. Store bought orange juice will have added ingredients where as an orange is a whole food, a natural food. It is healthier and better to eat foods without labels. Foods without labels are foods that come from a garden, a farmer's market, the produce aisle in a grocery store, farm raised, these are foods in their natural state.

If you drink soda or store-bought juice then you may want to start to cut back on how much you drink and how often you drink soda and store-bought juice. In the beginning it may be helpful to mix about three quarters soda and a quarter water to dilute it, same with the juice. If you can handle it, do half soda and half water or if you drink juice then do half juice and half water. It may be easier for you to slowly cut back on soda by adding water to it. It may change the taste and make you not like the diluted taste so you will quit the soda and juice quicker. Both soda and store-bought juice have a lot of sugar in them! I know how easy it is to be addicted to sugar, it is in everything. Marketing makes things sweet so we will like it and buy it. Remember, businesses do not care about your health, they want to make a sale and have you keep coming back as a customer.

Start eating the "rainbow of colors." Have you ever heard that before? It means to eat foods from many color groups. Eat the greens, blues, purples, reds, yellows, oranges, and whites. Start eating colorful foods. Colorful foods appeal to the eyes. Colorful foods make your plate pop. Foods just look more healthy and tasty better when they have color. Foods with color have more vitamins, nutrients and everything good for you. Fried foods, breaded foods, fast foods, and gravies are all of a brownish color. I am not sure about you, but I have never seen brownish colors in a rainbow. You will want to start reducing the amount of brown foods you put on your plate. Start reducing the number of times a day or week you have brown foods.

Reading labels is another great place to start. When you buy food with a label, read the label. First look to see if there are more than five ingredients in the food especially if your goal is to eat foods with five ingredients or less. Can you pronounce all the ingredients on the label? Do you know what all those ingredients are in the food you are about to buy? If there are more than five ingredients or if you cannot pronounce all those ingredients, do you want to be putting those ingredients into your body? After you read the ingredients list, look at how much sugar and sodium (salt) is in the food. Look for canned or frozen foods with the lowest sugar and lowest sodium to make the food healthier for you. Some things like donuts or muffins from the bakery do not have labels but that does not mean that you should be eating those items. When reading the label, is it one serving or two servings or more? If it is two or more servings, remember to double (or triple) the calories and everything else will then be doubled like fat, sugar, and sodium. How much protein does it have? Look at the vitamins listed, what you are about to eat, does it even have any nutritious value?

Another great place to start as you begin your healthy journey is to organize your pantry, countertop and refrigerator with healthy foods. As you learn more you will be buying and eating different foods which will be healthier foods. Ensure you have more fresh produce than processed boxed foods. Get rid of the canned foods that have high sodium content and high sugar content. It is healthier to cook fresh foods than to pour things out of a can all the time. Check the expiration dates and get rid of expired foods. If a can of food is badly dented, consider getting rid of that can because it may have a small hole in the can that you cannot see. Store dried goods in Mason jars or clear glass jars so you can see the contents of what is inside. Label your containers and remember to put the expiration date on the label. Do not keep junk foods and unhealthy foods visible on your countertops. If at all possible, do not even purchase junk food and bring it in the house. If you do not have junk food, you cannot be tempted to eat it. It is that simple. We eat with our eyes first and we will crave and eat what we see. Anything with ingredients that contain high fructose corn syrup, vegetable oil, artificial sweeteners and other such unhealthy ingredients are the items you will want to get rid of and start replacing with healthier foods.

Start looking for ways to add in more fruits and vegetables into your meals. A great way to do that is to eat a healthy salad or have a smoothie every day. Start small with maybe a small healthy side salad or maybe having a smoothie as a snack. As you get to liking salads or smoothies, start having a larger salad adding in more vegetables. Start adding in more vegetables into your smoothie and having it for breakfast instead of having it for a snack. It is better to have some vegetables in your diet than to have no vegetables in your diet.

Pull out your China and use it. You do not have to wait until a special occasion to use your China. You are the "special" occasion. Your health is special so celebrate by eating off your China. Treat yourself to a healthy salad on your China. Treat yourself to a smoothing using your fine crystal glasses. I say if you have China, start using it, do it for you!

When you wake up in the morning, unless you are truly going to be working out, start to get dressed in nicer clothes instead of workout clothing or lounging pants. When you start to dress nice, you feel better. When you dress in clothes that fit, bright colored clothes, you just feel better. I am sure you have heard it said before, "look good, feel good." Do not hide your body behind baggy clothing. Accept your body for what it is, it is your body from God. Treat it as such and take care of your body. Start waking up and getting dressed in clothing as if you were going to work, it does help you to feel better. When you feel better, you automatically feel healthier.

Start from my lessons learned so you do not have to make the same mistakes. Start now to get healthier so you do not waste as much time as I have to get healthy. Start now with the knowledge you will gain from reading this book.

You have to be honest to yourself. Do you want to get healthier and lose weight? Are you doing it for you or are you trying to do it for someone else? Are you serious about reaching your goals? Will you actually take the necessary steps to reach your goal of being healthier? If you say you will do such and such to reach your goal, will you? If you say you will do something, do it. Doing what you say you will do builds self-trust. If you are not going to do what you say, then subconsciously your mind knows that and will do everything to assure that you fail because you have not been true to yourself previously.

Say what you are going to do and do it because you have made yourself and your health a priority. Say it and do it and that will build self-trust and then you will reach your goals this time. Start and follow through with what you say you will do. You have to be able to trust yourself. You have to know when you say you will do something that you will actually do it. Develop that self-trust muscle same as you develop any muscle. The more you do what you say you will do, the more you develop that self-trust muscle.

You have to believe that you can do it, that you will be able to eat healthier and get healthier. This time will be different than any previous time that you tried because it is not a diet. You are going to learn to eat healthy for life this time. Do you believe you can do it? Believing that you can do it is a big part in doing it. Remain positive on your journey to eating healthier and you will be amazed at how simple it will be to eat healthy.

Start being more mindful of the things you say to yourself, the things you eat and the things you do. Just start being more mindful. Being mindful of the foods you are currently eating will help you to learn to make better food choices. Picture someone who you believe is a role model when it comes to eating healthy and notice the types of food they eat. Your role model is probably a picture of health. They eat healthy, they look healthy, and they are healthy. Start observing others when you go out and see what type of things they are eating or what type of things they are doing that could be impacting their health, whether impacting their health in a positive or negative way. Are they eating slowly? Do they smoke? Are they laughing and having a good time with family and friends? Just start noticing and being mindful of your choices. Are you yourself being a role model for others? When you are out, do you make healthy food choices since someone may be observing you?

If you are not already in the habit of saying a prayer to bless your food before you eat it, I encourage you to start that habit. A few seconds or a couple minutes that it takes helps you to be mindful, present, and helps to calm you down so you are not rushed when you eat. Being thankful for the food you are about to eat may help you to be more grateful in other areas of your life and not only with eating healthier foods.

When you begin to eat healthy and lose weight, you will gain more energy. I want you to be thinking of what losing weight and having more energy mean to you. Just imagine for a few minutes what losing weight will look like for you. Imagine having more energy to do the things you want to do. What are you going to do with yourself when you gain more energy? Write your visualization of losing weight and gaining energy in your journal. Refer back to your visualization often as to what losing weight and more energy looks like for you and it will help you to stay focused and on course on your healthy journey. When someone is asked why they want to lose weight, most often they say they want more energy. As you lose weight, you do gain more energy. As you eat healthy, you naturally lose weight and gain energy. As we move forward, be thinking what you are going to do with all your new energy that you will gain as you eat healthy. Another great place then to start with as you begin eating healthy is with your rising energy levels. You need to have a plan for your energy, how will you use your energy in a positive way?

I hope that you can see how simple all these ideas are to help you get started on your healthy journey. I want to keep things simple so you will start and stay the course to becoming healthy and healthier. The hard part is just starting, the simple part is eating healthy.

Will you be able to implement any or several of these simple ideas to get started? Maybe you are already doing a few of these things and that is awesome. Consider adding in different steps that I mentioned that you are not currently doing. Maybe you came up with a few of your own ideas as you were reading this chapter that will help you to start on your journey, and I strongly recommend you try your own ideas too. Write in your journal which ideas that I mentioned that you will start doing and which ones you would like to add in at a later time.

Do you feel you have anything standing in your way or holding you back from being successful at eating healthier? Let's move on to learning to "Let it Go".

Chapter 3

Let It Go

In this chapter, letting it go will be discussed. Maybe you are holding on to things that are preventing you from achieving your goals. What type of things could possibly be stopping you on your healthy journey?

Let's think about that for a moment. Do you think you are holding on to things that are preventing you from moving forward? Do you feel stuck? What type of things could you possibly be holding on to that is preventing you from being healthy?

In your mind, do you hear the voice of a parent, maybe a former spouse or current spouse, saying things like "you will never be good enough"? Or are you hearing your own voice saying things like "you were fat then and you will always be fat"? Whatever it is that you constantly hear, those negative self-sabotaging thoughts, let it go! It will be helpful to you to write down all the negative self-talk that you continue to say to yourself or that you hear in your head, and then throw it away. You can burn that piece of paper, you can shred what you wrote or you can rip it up and throw it away. Whatever you do, just let it go and get rid of that piece of paper with negative thoughts on it. No use holding on to that paper or holding on to those negative thoughts any longer than you already have. Let the burning, shredding, or throwing it away be a visual and reminder to you that your old, negative ways are gone and you are moving forward with a positive attitude to becoming a healthier you.

What about that incident that you view as a mistake that keeps coming back to your thoughts, like you had a piece of dessert at a picnic. It is not a mistake so stop beating yourself up. Let it go, you ate the dessert, accept it and move on. You do not have to feel as though it was mistake and now you will never be able to eat healthy.   That is so far from the truth and you need to let it go!

Maybe at one point in your life you were wronged by someone. No matter how severe the wrong to you, have you learned to forgive the person who wronged you? Forgiving the person does not mean you agree with what happened to you, or what was said to you, it just means that you are letting it go, forgiving that person and moving on. Forgiving is more about freeing your soul, giving you freedom and peace to not let that person or incident control you for the rest of your life. Forgiving is more about you and your attitude than about the other person. Forgive them. Please forgive them, do it for you, not for them.

Sometimes forgiveness is needed for what we said or done to someone else so we have to be able to forgive ourselves too. Once we say something, once those words slip off our tongue, it is too late to retrieve those words. The damage has been done, the words have been spoken. Now your words may have hurt someone else and scarred them for life. Now you need to forgive yourself so you can move forward. Let go of that guilt and shame that is causing you so much physical pain in the form of illness. Whatever you have done or said, to someone else or to yourself, please find it in your heart to forgive yourself.

What are you hiding that you need to bring to light and deal with? What shame do you have? These things that you have buried are now bringing stress and disease upon your body. These things may be causing you to overeat because you have never properly dealt with them. Maybe you do not know how to properly deal with these feelings and thoughts so you turn to food. Yet the very foods you are choosing to comfort you are actually the foods that are making you overweight and sick. Learn to let go of negative thoughts in a positive way.

When I think of "letting it go" I like to relate it with the old hymn, "It is Well with My Soul" written by Horatio G. Spafford in 1873. If something does not sit well with your soul, let it go, get rid of it and move on. My husband and I was involved in a program that took place twice a month for several years, and lately it seemed like the day before that program he would get tired, sick, run down, and grumpy. Then the morning of that program, we would be angry at each other and snapping, just basically hating life and taking it out on each other. After a few months of this happening, twice a month, I come to realize that it was not well with our souls. We needed to let it go and move on. If something is causing that much built up of tiredness, sickness, anger in our soul, we need to let it go. If something is no longer serving your soul and no longer has a purpose in your life, let it go.

Have you ever felt you were in a toxic relationship? Like that relationship was bringing you down, the person is always negative or making you negative and not helping you to be positive. I am not saying you have to leave your spouse or leave any relationship for that matter, I am just asking if you felt you were ever in a toxic relationship? Maybe you have friends that are always zapping the life out of you with their negativity or maybe at your place of employment there is negative energy there, all I am saying is you may want to think hard about letting it go if it does not sit well with your soul. Maybe changing the toxic relationship around into a positive relationship is all that needs to happen. I just want you to be in tune with your body and know when you need to let go and when you need to do a gut check to see if something is well with your soul. Toxic relationships may be causing you undo stress in your life which in turn may be making you overeat and be sick. It is your health that I care about.

I am sure you heard it said before to "clean out your closet". I say that figurative and literal, clean out your closet. What ghosts do you have lurking in your closet (your mind) that you could let go of so that you are living a healthier life? Our thoughts control our mood and our mood controls what we choose to eat, how much we choose to eat and if we will be choosing healthy foods to eat or not. If you are happy and positive you will choose healthier foods to eat. If you are upset, angry, holding on to stress, you are more likely going to be grabbing for unhealthy foods with the hope that the food will give you comfort.

In your closet of clothes, what are you holding on to that you know you can get rid of? Maybe you have lost weight and or inches in your body measurements, so why are you holding on to the clothes that are too large for you? To me, holding on to clothes that is too large for you is subconsciously giving yourself permission to gain the weight back. It is like you do not even trust yourself that you will succeed with eating healthy and you know you will gain the weight back one day so you hold on to those larger sized clothes. Let it go, get rid of the clothes that no longer fits you. You have come so far and you have lost the weight, be proud of it and wear clothes that fits. Stop wearing clothes that just hangs on you because you do not want to buy new clothes in a smaller size yet just in case you gain the weight back. You lost the weight and you should be proud of it. Clean out your closet! Let it go.

Same with holding on to clothes that are too small for you in hopes you will one day lose the weight and fit back into those clothes. Let it go and when you lose the weight, reward yourself with new clothes that fits. What if while holding on to clothes that you hope to fit back into the style changes? Are you still going to want to wear those smaller sizes? Probably not, so let it go and get rid of it. As you lose the weight, reward yourself for reaching your mini goals and buy a few pieces of new clothes.

It is not just your clothes closet that need to be cleaned out. Why are you holding on to things in your house that no longer serve you? Clutter and holding on to material things could be an indication that you are holding on to other things, things inside of you that you need to let go of. Once you let go of the clutter inside of you then the clutter outside of you (things in your house causing clutter) will be gone too. The opposite is true also, if you start to let go of the material things and clutter that no longer is needed, then the clutter inside of you leaves you too.   Cleaning house, inside your physical body and inside your physical house, are very healing. Eating healthy helps you to heal same as cleaning the clutter helps you to heal. Clutter will make you depressed, drained, no energy, and cause you to eat poorly and be unhealthy. If you have clutter you probably are not living a simply life. You may feel you need more and more material things and then that attitude drains over into your eating habits, always wanting more and more to eat.

What about the mirror or the bathroom scale, do you need to let go of them? Are they helping you become healthier or are they making you become more depressed? If you are able to look in the mirror and love who is looking back at you, then by all means, keep looking in the mirror. Are you are using a mirror but treating it like a magnifying mirror to look at yourself? I can promise you that no one looks at you as closely as you look at yourself. Why are you critiquing yourself under a magnifying mirror? Why are you critiquing yourself to that detail? If you are looking at yourself in a full-length mirror, it needs to be to see if your clothing matches and not to judge your body appearance. Are you more positive when you look in your mirrors or more negative? Same with the bathroom scale, is it your friend or not? I believe that your health, your mood, your journal, and your clothes fitting loser are all great indicators whether you are losing weight and you may not even need the bathroom scale. If you do not need the bathroom scale, get rid of it. If the mirror and bathroom scale are not well with your soul, let them go!

Let go of your old ways of eating. You have to let go of your old ways of eating and let go of the foods that are no longer serving you well. Let go of fried food, fast food, desserts, and junk food. Let it go! Do not look back, let it go! Marketing only wants your money so they want you to like their foods. Marketing does not care about your health. Let go of your old ways of eating. Just let it go! When you are eating anything, ask yourself how important is it for you to be healthy? Is what you are eating helping you to become healthier or not? If your health is important to you, start to make better, healthier food choices. Let go of your old way of eating. Be open to trying new foods and healthier foods. Remember, if you always do what you have always done you will always get the same results. You have to let go of the old foods and start eating new, healthy foods. The healthier you eat, the more you will like healthier foods. Your taste buds do change so you will be liking and craving healthier foods soon. Remember your goal, what is your goal? Was your goal to eat healthy to be healthy? I do not know anyone who has ever regretted eating better, having more energy from eating healthier and regretted feeling worse when they were feeling healthier.

Let go of your old way of thinking. Let go of thinking that you know how to eat healthy and be open to learning new ways of eating. Let go of thinking what you are doing is working for you when in reality it probably is not working for you. Let go of that thought that you always have done it this way, it is familiar to you and so you want to continue that way of eating. Maybe your old way of thinking is that you need milk for calcium or you need dessert all the time. Both of those statements are so far from the truth it is unreal.

Another way to let go of things is to give yourself permission to let go. You may think you have to always eat the same way, the same foods and do the same things because that is what you know and was taught to do. If you just tell yourself you will be doing things differently, trying new things, letting go of the old ways, then you are giving yourself permission to shake things up. It is a way of letting go when you give yourself permission to do it.

I think another thing about letting it go is that you have to be really honest with yourself. You have to be transparent with yourself and be real with yourself. You have to ask yourself those hard questions, like "do you really want to eat healthier?" Maybe you say you want to eat healthier but then when it comes down to it, maybe you do not want to eat healthier because you fear that your family or friends will not invite you over to eat because you are eating healthier. Just that negative thought will stop you dead in your tracks from really wanting to eat healthier. You have to let go of fear. Do not fear and worry about what others will think about you now that you are eating healthier. Eat healthy anyway and do it for you. Do not fear that you will not lose the weight. If you are eating healthier, you will lose the weight. Do not fear that you will not know what to eat that is healthy. You will learn which foods are the healthier option as you go along on your journey. Do not let fear control you! Let go of fear and do it anyway.

Another thing about "Let it Go" is I love when I see those inflatable air dancers, (things at a car dealer to draw your attention to a sale) flopping in the air like dancing. When I visualize letting it go, I visualize that air dancer flopping his arms and dancing about. He is happy, letting it go, not a worry in the world. He is celebrating his new life, free from all the pain, free from all the clutter. Just let it go so you can dance around with that same freedom. Also seeing those inflatable air dancers makes me just want to let it go, dance as if no one is watching. Be happy, get into it, let it go, have fun! Letting it go does not have to be a negative experience that you are letting go of, it could be to let go, have fun, do not be so hard on yourself. Dance around, let it go, be you, celebrate you and who you are becoming.

It seems all the choices we make in life can affect what we eat and what we put on our plate. If you are making healthy choices, you are more likely to be eating healthier. It all comes full circle, think of it like a plate, a circle. What we think does affects what we eat. What we hold on to affects what we eat. When you are stressed you may eat differently than when you are not stressed. What we eat affects how we feel. It all comes full circle and the choices we make in life comes back to our plate and therefore to our health. Therefore, be careful what foods you put on your plate and be careful what you do and think because it affects what foods you put on your plate.

Can you see how things you may be holding on to may be preventing you from achieving your goal of being healthy? What can you start to let go of today that will help you as you move forward to being your healthiest self? Do you have any "baggage" you need to get rid of?

Up until this point, everything has been to help you get started on your healthy journey. Now I am going to be real transparent and tell you what healthy is for me and the things I eat and do to be healthy. Are you ready to hear how I cleaned up my eating and what foods I eat?

Chapter 4

Foods I Eat

I have mentioned eat healthy to be healthy and now I will show you what eating healthy looks like. I will share with you the type of foods I eat. I have slowly altered and modified the foods I used to eat to the healthy foods I eat now. I will mention healthy foods and since you are now being open to trying new foods, I suggest you try eating these healthier foods.

Some ingredients we just know should not be in our foods let alone in our bodies if we are trying to eat healthy. I immediately cut out anything containing high fructose corn syrup (ketchup, sodas, candy, breakfast cereals, salad dressings and sweetened yogurts). There are many foods with high fructose corn syrup as one of the listed ingredients so be careful what you eat. It is important you read labels for that reason so you are not putting things in your body that are harmful to your body.

I threw out my vegetable oil and switched to using extra virgin olive oil. I used to use vegetable oil only for baking and I hardly ever bake now. When I do bake I look for healthier recipes that use healthier oils, unsweetened apple sauce or avocados, almond flour instead of white flour, and recipes that use less sugar. When I bake, I bake things from scratch and not a box mix.

You can use vegetable broth instead of extra virgin olive oil when sautéing foods making it even healthier and it may even add a little extra flavor. Use olives on your salads instead of using olive oil as olives are in their natural state. I do use extra virgin olive oil for cooking and as a base for salad dressing, as we need healthy fats in our diets. I am not against extra virgin olive oil and in moderation it is okay.

I stopped using artificial sweeteners in my coffee. I stopped drinking all those fancy coffee drinks with all those calories. I now drink organic black coffee, or green tea or healthy lattes with unsweetened almond milk or unsweetened coconut milk. I drink a lot more water than I used to drink. I hardly ever drank sodas but I definitely do not drink sodas now.

My husband and I make our own distilled water, yogurt, and unsweetened almond milk. Distilled water is the best water you can drink. You can buy distilled water in grocery stores and we did for years but it comes in plastic gallon jugs. If you are going to be drinking the best water do you really want to be buying it in plastic gallon jugs? We make our distilled water in glass jars. Our tap water is so hard and filled with so many chemicals that it leaves water marks on everything including our coffee pot. Now with using distilled water the coffee pot does not have water marks. Water, coffee and foods we make using distilled water just tastes better and cleaner. We buy a plain Greek yogurt and then make our own plain yogurt straining out most of the whey through a nut bag.

This is how I make my unsweetened almond milk. I buy raw whole almonds. Using a small Mason jar or small container that has a lid, soak one cup of almonds in just enough water to cover the almonds. Put the container in the refrigerator overnight or up to a few days. Drain the water and rinse the almonds. Measure out 3 to 4 cups of cold distilled water. Put part of the almonds in a Nutri Bullet and blend for about one minute. Pour this almond mixture through a nut bag that is over a glass jar. I continue blending almonds and water until all the almonds and distilled water are used up. Let that drip through the nut bag and then twist and wring the nut bag over the jar getting out all the water. I throw away the almond pulp but you could leave that in your milk if you want. There you have it, homemade unsweetened almond milk! You can use less or more water to your liking. You can use a little salt, but you do not have to. You can leave the pulp in and not strain it out or leave some pulp in. If you want it sweetened, you can blend in a couple pitted Medjool dates with the almonds and water. If you want, you can add in a little cinnamon or a little vanilla extract or both. Experiment to see what mixture you like best. There are many different recipes on the internet for making your own almond milk so you can choose the one that you like best.

I do not eat breakfast cereals anymore. A lot of the breakfast cereals are made with white flours and have lots of added sugars. I eat steel cut oatmeal or old fashioned rolled oats. Instead of always eating oatmeal, brown rice is a great substitute because the color, texture and taste are about the same. I use brown rice as my oatmeal on some days. I eat cooked, warm oatmeal or old fashioned rolled oats soaked in alternative milk for about 10 minutes to soften. Sometimes I add fruit, nuts, seeds, cinnamon, honey or alternative milk to my oatmeal and sometimes I just eat it warm and plain. Sometimes I add cacao powder or carob powder to my oatmeal if I want something chocolatey. I do not eat oatmeal every morning. Eating too much grains causes inflammation in our body. I noticed eating too much grains makes my joints stiff.

I do not eat white pasta and all those pasta sauces. I use sprouted grain pasta and will either put extra virgin olive oil with diced fresh tomatoes and fresh or dry herbs on top or I will use a sauce that has the least amount of sugar. I do like brown rice pasta, brown rice or quinoa as my pasta. Pasta should be eaten as a side and not the main meal especially if using regular white flour pasta.

I drink a lot more smoothies now than I ever did. Smoothies are a great way to get in your nutrients, vitamins, and get different fruit and vegetables into your diet. Smoothies can be made with water, alternative milks, yogurt, coconut water, even juicy fruits for the liquid in the smoothie. Add in whatever vegetables you have on hand, add in a fruit or two and you have a smoothie. You can add in nuts, seeds, protein powders, basically you can add pretty much anything you like and have on hand. I remember the first time I ever ordered a smoothie out in public and they asked me if I wanted water or sugar water added to my smoothie. I was surprised that they would take a healthy smoothie and even think of adding sugar water to it. Often times when someone thinks of a smoothie, they think of strawberry, banana, milk and maybe yogurt. That type of smoothie is more of a milkshake because of the natural sugars than a healthy smoothie. Smoothies are a great way to disguise vegetables to get you and your family to eat that vegetable. I like to use a 3 to 1 ratio when making smoothies, 3 vegetables to 1 fruit.

Have you heard of a smoothie bowl? Smoothie bowls are basically a smoothie poured into a bowl and then toppings are added so you eat your smoothie instead of drinking your smoothie. A smoothie bowl helps you practice mindful eating since you have to sit, eat and chew. To me a smoothie bowl can be yogurt, then your fruit on top, add other things like flax seed, nuts, chia seeds, or even add cacao or cooked oatmeal. Whatever you like in your smoothie you will like on your smoothie bowl. You can blend a smoothie without adding all the ingredients, pour it in a bowl, then add sliced banana on top, there is your smoothie bowl. I also like to make oatmeal and instead of having a cup of fruit next to my oatmeal, I add it on top, add a dollop of plain yogurt and there is my smoothie bowl.

I do like plain Greek yogurt and plain whole milk Kiefer for the taste and for their probiotic benefits. I keep trying to cut out dairy so I am drinking more Kombucha for the probiotic benefits. If you are lactose intolerant, usually you can drink Kiefer with no problem. Other healthy probiotics that you could eat if you do not like Greek yogurt or yogurt are Kiefer, Kombucha, sauerkraut or kimchi. If you are going to buy sauerkraut, buy homemade sauerkraut as it has less sugar. If you had to take antibiotics at any time in your life, then your stomach gut flora has changed and you may want to be eating more probiotic foods to get your gut flora corrected.

If you like plain Greek yogurt in your smoothie, have you tried using plain Kiefer instead? You have to get used to both tastes, Greek yogurt and Kiefer. Start with a small amount of plain Greek yogurt or Kiefer mixed in your smoothie and as you get used to the taste over a few weeks then keep adding in more. I sometimes have a smoothie bowl with Kiefer instead of using Greek yogurt. I pour Kiefer in a bowl, add blueberries and halved seedless grapes to the bowl and eat with a spoon or blend it up and drink it as a smoothie.   Probiotics and antioxidants, cannot go wrong with adding these into your daily eating to help support healthy digestion.

I eat green leafy salads now. Often times when we eat out, I decide where to go by which restaurant serves a salad using any leafy green other than choosing a restaurant that only uses iceberg lettuce. I like restaurants that have a nice salad bar. I often order salads now when we eat out, unlike before my healthy journey where I would order unhealthy meals. Be careful eating at salad bars. Just because an item is on a salad bar or comes in a salad does not mean it is a healthy option. A lot of times at salad places or on a salad that you order, you will see dried cranberries, candied walnuts, cheeses, salad dressings already on your salad and even croutons or pita bread served with your salad. These are not the healthiest items to be putting on your salads. I order salads with a lot of cut up fresh or maybe roasted vegetables, maybe diced fruit, and salad dressing on the side. I rarely use salad dressings on my salads especially in a restaurant.

I love to read recipes and look at the beautiful pictures of recipes. I also love to read a recipe and see if I can make it healthier than it is. To me, some ingredients in recipes are interchangeable. Of course, that all depends on what you are making if you can switch up the ingredients. Do you look at a recipe and follow it precisely or do you like to use recipes as a guide and add your own twist to the recipe?   I usually follow the recipe exactly the first time to try it then I alter it the next time I make it. I will write a note on the recipe if it had too much salt or was bland or too spicy or whatever and then the next time I make it to my liking. To me, recipes are a guide, a suggestion to do things a certain way and they can be altered to your liking. Experiment and try different recipes and alter them to your tastes. It is fun!

I do not order desserts now when I eat out. That was a very hard habit for me to break, but I broke that habit! You will be able to break that habit too one day. Look at desserts as your enemy and not your friend, because that is really what dessert is. Do not look at desserts as a treat, like you are treating yourself or rewarding yourself. When you do eat desserts, it is actually punishing yourself. When I used to give in to ordering desserts, then I would feel guilty, upset, angry, fat and even bloated. Is that really the way I want to feel when I eat something? If I do not order dessert, then I do not have to deal with those negative feelings and thoughts. Have you ever noticed in restaurants that they seem to always walk you past the desserts before seating you? That is marketing at its finest, sending a subliminal message to get you craving the desserts even before you eat your meal.

I eat a lot of raw vegetables now. Vegetables do not always have to be boiled, steamed, roasted or cooked to enjoy them. I like to eat raw vegetables and enjoy their natural flavor, crunch and texture. Do not be hesitant to try different fruits and vegetables. The worse that could happen is you will not like them at first or maybe the worst is that you will like new fruits and vegetables and have to buy them more often. Remember half your plate each meal should be vegetables, preferably non-starchy vegetables.

Don't you wish back then that you knew what you know now about eating healthy? Hindsight really is 20/20.

Chapter 5

Hindsight really is 20/20

When I was growing up, I do not remember ever hearing about all this food craze-- organic food, probiotics, supplements, combining certain foods for better absorption, or anything remotely close to all of this. Growing up I did not know about portion size or counting calories. I did not know about reading food labels. I did not know which foods were healthy for me and which foods were processed. I just ate and did not think about any of these things. I was not taught how to eat healthy. Eating healthy was something I had to learn on my own over the years. Like most of you, you were probably not taught to eat healthy either, and it was something you also had to learn for yourself over the years. I did not know that what I ate would affect my health or my skin.   In hindsight, I wish I would have known about these things and other things to help me to be healthier now. I am telling you though that it is never too late to start taking care of yourself and your health. Maybe you did not learn anything about being healthy when you were younger and that is okay. It is never too late to start eating healthy. Do not beat yourself up for what you did not learn when you were younger about eating healthy and just be happy you are learning to eat healthy now. Things that I wish I knew then that I know now are the things I am going to share with you. It is amazing, in hindsight we are all so much smarter.

Back to the time I was in the military, starting as early as basic training, there is so much now that I wished I knew back then. I'm glad I learned to eat vegetables but I wish I would have known how good vegetables were for me and not only eat them because I was afraid of my drill sergeants. I ate so fast in basic training and I know now that was not good for my digestion to eat that fast. I was not being mindful when I ate. I never even heard of mindful eating when I was in the military and I think that is what the military would have called an oxymoron. Could you imagine being in the military and practicing mindful eating? I could imagine it now and it makes me laugh, "Oh drill sergeant, I am not finished eating, could I get 15 more minutes so I can chew my food slower and longer?" Yeah, that would have went over really well! I could barely taste my food since I ate so fast let alone notice the texture of my food. I did not chew my food long enough to begin breaking down my food to aid with digestion. I did not eat until I was 80% full then stop eating. I ate until I was full each and every time I ate. I know now that I cannot "treat" myself to pizza every Friday night and eat leftover pizza all weekend. I have learned that it is not a "treat" to buy food for myself, especially unhealthy food. A treat or a reward should be something like new clothing or a manicure and not treat myself with unhealthy food. Like I stated before, while I was in the military, I sure wish I would have known that you cannot exercise your way out of a bad diet. It is better to have learned it now than to not have learned it at all.

Another goal of mine is to have clear, glowing skin. In hindsight, I had no idea what I ate affected my skin. Who knew? One way to have great skin is by what you eat. This is another great reason why it is so important to eat healthy. What goes in must come out, whether it comes out as healthy skin or unhealthy skin, what you eat comes out. The foods you eat may either come out as sickness or maybe as a model of health. I know with a goal of wanting clear, glowing skin, that goal alone helps me to eat healthier foods. Ensure you are putting healthy foods into your body so your skin will be vibrant. Your skin is your body's first tattle tell sign as to whether you are eating healthy or not. When you are hydrated your skin just looks better and healthier. If you are eating a lot of junk foods, fried foods, unhealthy foods, it will reflect in your skin. Your skin reflects what you eat as does your health reflect what you eat.

I was always a very gassy person, and I thought that was just the way of life for everyone. I did not question it, I had no reason to. I ate, I would get gas, such is life. I had no idea that diet and the foods we ate could cause one person to be gassy and not another person. I mean consuming diary made me real gassy. Other foods that commonly give someone gas are onions, beans, and broccoli. I had no idea that when I ate things with cow's milk, like drinking a glass of milk, having a bowl of cereal, a piece of cheese or eating ice cream that it caused me to have severe stomach pains and gas. Once I learned how bad dairy was for me, I immediately switched to using alternative milks. I commonly buy unsweetened almond milk or make my own unsweetened almond milk. I do buy unsweetened coconut milk too. I had ice cream a few times this summer and each time I was bent over in so much pain in my stomach it was unreal. I realized it is no longer worth it to me to eat ice cream if dairy puts me in that much pain and discomfort. I no longer care to eat or crave ice cream and dairy products.

To get rid of one habit you have to replace it with a new habit. Who knew that? I thought just stop the bad habit that no longer serves you. But I realized it does helps to stop a bad habit when it is replaced with a new, good habit. Get rid of the old ways of doing things, the old way of thinking and replace that old habit with a new healthier habit. First, this would have meant that I would have to be aware of and recognize that I had an old habit to break. I wish earlier in life that I would have recognized my bad eating habits and replaced my bad eating habits with clean eating habits. I am telling you that it is never too late to start eating healthy. Okay, so I did not recognize that I had bad eating habits prior to a couple years ago, but once I learned of my bad eating habits, I started making modifications to my eating habits. It was that simple, once I knew a food was bad for me, I learned to replace it with good food.

Another goal of mine is to eat foods with 5 ingredients or less. This is a goal of mine and am I not always able to do this but I am eating cleaner and healthier than I ever ate. I told someone once that I try to eat foods with 5 ingredients or less and they said "tell me those 5 ingredients and I will eat them." It is not a certain "5 ingredients" but rather it is eating foods that have 5 ingredients or less. Eating foods with 5 ingredients or less means you are eating more whole foods, eating more plant based foods, eating foods without labels and eating foods that are less processed. Like I said before, I never used to read food labels. I had no idea I even had to read labels if I wanted to eat healthier. In hindsight, I had no idea what ingredients were lurking in our foods. I had no idea how muc

h sugar, chemicals and other things are added in our food. I had no idea when you buy foods like coconut chips (which is dried coconut pieces) they add sugar to something that already is sweet on its own.

I really wish I would have known that holding on to clutter and "things" meant that I may also hold on to my weight. Who knew! It all makes sense, because you are holding on to something. I wish I learned at an earlier age that clutter is bad for your weight let alone the common things that clutter does such as look cluttered, make you depressed and of course not being able to breath with all that dust on the clutter.

In hindsight, I know now that I had to quit preparing to be ready one day and just make today the day. I had to just start and do it. I could not just sit on the couch and wish I had a better body, healthier body or that I weighed less, I had to actually do something for it to become reality. No wishing, I had to do it. I had to start and continue to make healthy swaps of foods so I would be eating healthier.

Continue to eat healthy and do not give up and it will work for you. Everything in this book has worked for me, is working for me and it will work for you too. Want to know what specifically worked for me?

Chapter 6

It Worked for Me

I know you want to know specifically what I ate that cured my thyroid issues, and specifically what I ate that helped me to lose weight. I know you want to know what I ate that gave me more energy and also helped me to sleep better. You want to know what gave me better health overall. Well, I cannot tell you one specific food cured me of my thyroid issues. I cannot even tell you specifically one food that helped me lose weight. I can however tell you that it was a combination of everything in this book that helped me. It would be easier if I told you the foods I cut out of my diet that allowed me to be healthier. I will tell you what I believed helped me the most.

I had to just do it. I had to stop planning to be ready and just know I was ready and to just start. I had to stop preparing to be ready and just start. I had to stop saying next week on Monday I will start. I had to just start, regardless of what day it was that day and just start. I realized I did not need every workout DVD before I started. I realized I did not need a lot of work out clothing before I started. It was more important that I just start. No more excuses and no more procrastination, I had to just do it, just start and go forward from there. Once I started I had to continue so I would see and feel the results of eating healthy. It was like I knew I could not turn back now, I had to keep moving forward and continue making healthier decisions.

I had to believe that what I was doing was important for me and my overall health. If I did not feel it was important, then I probably would have stopped shortly after I started down my healthy journey. I had to believe I was making the proper food choices. I had to know what I was doing was making a difference in my weight, my body and in my overall health. I had to be doing it for me, getting healthy for me and not for anyone else.

I can tell you I had to change my attitude toward eating and toward exercise. I had to be open to trying new and different foods which were healthier foods than what I was eating. I had to view exercise differently. I would walk my dog every day, rain or shine, anywhere from 1 to 3 to 6 miles a day. I kept saying "I really need to exercise, all I do is walk my dog." When I started viewing walking my dog as exercise instead of just viewing walking him as a means for him to go the bathroom, then I started appreciating walking and realized it is great exercise. If I did other exercise above walking my dog 3 to 6 miles a day, then great. If I only walked him and did no other exercise, then great, at least I was exercising and moving every day. But I had to change my attitude about exercise because I never used to view walking or walking my dog as exercise, now I know walking is great exercise. First, I had to change my attitude about exercise. When I changed my thinking about walking my dog, I then begin looking forward to walking him. Walking my dog was my exercise. I was not just walking him until he went the bathroom, we both were walking for exercise. Sometimes we would walk, sometimes we would run, and sometimes we would do both. Walking or walking your dog is exercise my friend. Exercise does not have to be lifting weights or going to a gym for it to be exercise. Walking my dog 3 to 6 miles a day toned my legs.

When I would receive a compliment from someone, that made me want to keep doing my healthy eating. When my doctor said to me "I'm not sure what you are doing, but keep doing it" and "Your numbers look great and you look great," then I knew I was doing the right thing by eating healthy. My clothes are fitting loser, I have increased energy, and I feel great. I do not need compliments because I know that eating healthy is the key to being healthy. Eating healthy is working for me. Compliments are great because it lets me know that others are seeing the results of me eating healthy. Compliments just make me want to continue forward with eating healthy and to do even more so I get more compliments. It is a win-win cycle, the better I eat, the more others compliment me and the more they complement me the more I want to eat healthy.

I cut out all those sugary coffee drinks that I used to have almost daily or a couple times a day. Now I will have a coffee latte on a rare occasion but it is made with coconut milk or almond milk and no cool whip on top. My coffee lattes are less sugary now and I have them a lot less often.

I cut out dairy. I either make or buy my own unsweetened almond milk or buy unsweetened coconut milk.

I cut out breads almost totally from my diet. Occasionally I will have a piece of sprouted grain bread. Pizza is like a once or twice a year meal now due to all that crust which is bread from white flour. Remember pizza used to be my every Friday go-to meal for years. If I order a hamburger, I will either order it bun less or just eat the bottom bun and not both buns. When I have a hamburger at home, I always eat it without a bun. I no longer use ketchup or barbeque sauce due to all the sugars in those condiments.

I used to drench my salads with salad dressing. Now I can eat salads without dressings because I enjoy the taste of the vegetables in my salad. I use apple cider vinegar and extra virgin olive oil often for my dressing. Sometimes I use 1-2 tablespoons of hummus as my dressing or hummus with extra virgin olive oil as a creamy dressing. I like to use salsa as my salad dressing, too. Salsa is one of those things that is so easy to make and can be whatever ingredients you like in your salsa. Sometimes the ingredients you put in your salad, when you cut it all up into same size pieces, it makes its own juice which is why I can eat salads plain without dressing. A fresh squeezed lemon over a salad makes a nice treat too.

Speaking of salsa, I like to look at the ingredients listed on a salsa that I am thinking of buying, then go buy those ingredients and I make my own salsa. If a jar of salsa lists ingredients such as tomatoes, onions, green pepper, salt, onion powder and garlic powder then I would buy those ingredients and make my own salsa. I would use onion and not onion powder since onion is a real, whole food. I would use garlic instead of garlic powder since garlic is healthier for you since it is less processed than garlic powder. I would purchase fresh garlic and not jarred garlic since that has preservatives. That is what I do, I read labels and try to make it myself at home instead of buying it. I do this not only with salsa but with everything. I read the ingredients list and try to make it instead of buying and eating processed or packaged foods.

I eat a lot more avocados than I ever used to eat. I love avocados! They are so good for you and so versatile! You can do everything with avocados from using it as a butter on your toast to even eating it as a snack to using it as a salad topping. You can eat avocados plain, with a little salt, with balsamic vinaigrette or even with a hard-boiled egg. Diced tomatoes with diced avocados tastes absolutely awesome and even more delicious with chopped fresh cilantro added! I make my own guacamole. Guacamole could be just smashed avocado or add in whatever you like in your guacamole like diced tomatoes, finely shredded leafy greens, spices, and a little fresh squeezed lemon or lime. Be creative, not only with avocados but with all fruits, vegetables, and whole foods to see what you will like.

I do not use any artificial sweeteners. I do add honey to a few things but I do not always have to add honey. Sometimes with my hot tea or oatmeal I like to add a bit of honey.

I read labels and I do not use anything with high fructose corn syrup in it. I cut out ketchup and that was hard because I used to use ketchup on a lot of different meats.

Walking my dog at least 3 times a day for at least one mile each time really helped me to tone my legs.   Even if you do not have a dog, you can still get out and walk three times a day and walk a mile each time.

Using a tracking device to monitor my steps really helped me too. I would compete against my own tracking device.   When my tracking device said I needed like 800 more steps to reach my daily goal of 10,000 steps, I would walk 900 more steps just to be ahead of my daily step goal. I made it a game with my tracking device. When my tracking device would say I needed to get up and move to finish the hour strong, I would walk around the block even though I only needed a few steps for that hour. My dog and I would walk, for my health and not because he had to go the bathroom. He never seemed to mind going for a walk with me.

When I work out, I want to eat better. When I eat better, it makes me want to work out. Together, working out and eating healthy, are a win-win situation. Cannot go wrong with working out and eating healthy so do them simultaneously. When you eat healthy, you have energy to work out. When you work out, you feel good about yourself so you want to eat healthy. After you work out, you want to eat healthy therefore not wasting all the effort of working out on a bad diet. It is a cycle, when you eat healthy, you want to work out and take care of your body. When you work out, you want to eat well, and so the cycle begins. When you eat poorly, you feel sluggish, guilty, lazy, then you do not work out. The next thing you know, years has gone by and you did not work out and you did not change your eating.

Drinking more water definitely helped me. Water gave me more energy while flushing out my toxins. It gave me clearer skin. Water helped me not to be hungry. Drinking water prevented me from drinking all those sugary coffee drinks that I used to drink. Now I drink water throughout the day.   I used to drink water mainly at meal time.

Drinking apple cider vinegar has helped me too. Apple cider vinegar gives me energy. I feel as though I am healing from the inside out when I drink apple cider vinegar. It is beneficial for everyone to drink apple cider vinegar. After drinking an apple cider vinegar drink it makes it harder to eat poorly knowing I just drank something good for me. Apple cider vinegar does help with digestion.

I always want to set a positive example and be a role model to others to eat healthy to be healthy. Just wanting to set a positive example as a health coach keeps me wanting to eat healthy. I always want people to catch me doing the right thing. I want to be eating healthy when they see me in a restaurant. I want to be outside working out so when people see me working out hopefully I am influencing and motivating them to work out.

I have heard a lot of women say it is harder to lose weight after entering menopause so I wanted to be as healthy and fit as possible going into menopause. I did not want to worry about gaining weight during menopause. I knew I needed to be in good eating habits prior to menopause. I wanted to set myself up for success so I started eating healthy a few years before menopause. The funny thing, I have toned more and lost more weight while in menopause then prior to menopause. I am proof that you can lose weight while in menopause, it can be done.

Having an attitude of gratitude, and just viewing things differently has been really helpful for me. Whether you write three positives or three things you are grateful for before bed or whenever you write your three things, it does help you to be more grateful. Writing the things you are grateful for keeps you more focused on things to be grateful for. It almost is like it keeps you more aware, more alert to watching for things to be grateful for. It changes your attitude from negative to positive when you are keeping track of the positives in your life. If you are having a bad day, stop and immediately write three things you are grateful for and see how quickly your attitude is turned around. It works for me.

I have always liked to read recipes, collect recipes and buy all kinds of recipe cook books and magazines. I even enjoy buying exercise books and magazines. There came a time when I said enough is enough. I had to use what I had and just know that I had enough. It finally hit me one day that reading all the recipe books in the world and reading all the exercise books was not going to change me. I had to just step out on faith that I knew enough, I have enough recipes, I have enough knowledge on how to exercise and just step out and do it. I had to quit reading and start doing. Putting into practice what I read, recipes or exercises, is what I began doing. I sometimes laugh because all the time I spent buying, collecting, reading those books I could have been "doing" something useful like making a healthy dish or exercising instead of just reading about it. Buying and reading these type books and magazines is not a bad thing, in fact, it may keep you focused and motivated to stay the course of eating healthy. There came a time for me when I had to say enough is enough and I had to just implement everything I had read.

View each new day as just that, a new day, a fresh start with new opportunities. Do not wait for the New Year to begin again or for a fresh start. Do not think "well, I blew it this year with my eating so I might as while wait until next year to start." That is the wrong attitude. I view each time I eat as a new opportunity to eat healthy and make the healthiest choices. I do not even need to wait until tomorrow to start fresh, I can start today, right now and so can you. I did not wait until tomorrow or next year, I started right now, right where I was to make better food choices and eat healthier.

I really had to be honest with myself and I had to ask myself all those hard questions. I asked myself questions like, "Are you happy with yourself?" "Do you love yourself?" and "Do you like what you see in the mirror?" If I could not answer those questions or answer them honestly, then I was never going to get anywhere until I was honest with myself. I had to ask myself if I really wanted change and if so, what was holding me back.

Mantras helps me. I repeat over and over to myself in my head "If you always do what you have always done you will always get the same results." Another one that helps me is "You can have results or excuses, not both, which will it be?" Also, another favorite mantra of mine is "You go girl, you can do it!" These are what worked for me to keep me motivated and on track with eating healthy and working out.

Have you ever felt there are things your doctor has never discussed with you but probably should discuss with you? In that case, I am going to discuss some things with you that you need to know while on your healthy journey.

Chapter 7

Doctors Won't Tell You, But I Will

Doctors will not tell you but you need to know is what this chapter is all about. Doctors may not tell you but I am going to tell you. This chapter will include a lot of information that affects your overall health and may not necessarily be about the foods you eat. Doctors do not have the time to sit with you for one hour, each visit, and tell you the things you need to eat or do to be your healthiest. Most doctor appointments are not even one hour long unless maybe it is your annual visit. Your doctor may say "you could lose some weight" or may say "it would be helpful to you if you cut out salt" but your doctor is not going to tell you how to do these things. If you lost weight and you tell your doctor you lost weight, your doctor may say "great, I wanted you to lose some weight." Your doctor is not going to discuss with you what you did to lose the weight, or find out what worked for you. Your doctor will just be happy you lost some weight. Whereas I as a Certified Health Coach will spend time with you and discuss with you how to eat healthier and give ideas, suggestions and recommendations to help you along on your journey. As a Certified Health Coach, I am going to ask you how you lost the weight, how you are feeling now that you lost some weight, and what type things will you do moving forward to keep the weight off.

Some of the things in this chapter will be basic steps you can take toward your overall health. Maybe you are already doing some of these ideas or taking these steps to have overall better health, if not maybe you can start including some of these ideas into your day-to-day life.

A very simple thing that you can do every day that will help you feel better is to make your bed every morning. I know you are wondering how does making your bed first thing every morning help you to be healthier. The moment we wake up we are preparing ourselves for a good night's rest. It feels so good at night to get in bed and the bed is made, the sheets and blankets are laying just right and in the same direction. When you get in a bed that has not yet been made, the sheets are not laying straight, they may be half off the bed and it just never feels right and you cannot get comfortable. But if you made your bed the first thing in the morning, it is done. You begin your day happier and it seems as though everything else in your day just seems to fall into place. It is a great feeling to know you have already accomplished one thing today. Your doctor is not going to tell you to make your bed every morning. Yet it is one thing that you can do every day that will help you to feel better.

Dental hygiene is another thing that you may be asking how can that help you to be healthier. Well, it does. Brushing your teeth, flossing and gargling are all great ways of getting germs and toxins out of your body. But have you ever thought to add oil pulling to your daily dental hygiene? Using a liquid oil like coconut oil, swish it around in your mouth to remove more germs and toxins from your body. Swish the oil around anywhere from 5 minutes to 20 minutes. You can do this swishing as you are in the shower or even as you are making your bed. Spit the oil in a disposable cup and throw it away. Do not spit the oil in your sink as it will eventually clog your drains. I recently read that doing oil pulling helps with so many diseases even arthritis because you are removing the toxins from your body. It cannot hurt to add it to your daily dental hygiene. Do you use a tongue scraper on a daily basis to get rid of any remaining foods on your tongue? Those remaining foods on your tongue could be causing your cravings and causing you to eat when you are not hungry. On occasion, I brush my teeth with peroxide or a little baking soda to naturally keep my teeth white. I use a natural toothpaste without added fluoride and I always use a soft bristle toothbrush. I gargle with apple cider vinegar and I use apple cider vinegar mixed with a little water to rinse my mouth with after oil pulling. Again, dental hygiene is one of these basic steps that you are probably already in the habit of doing daily and did not realize how important it is to your overall health. Maybe you have not yet started working oil pulling into your morning dental hygiene so this is something you could experiment with to see if you will like it and continue doing for life.

Does your doctor talk to you about deodorant and anti-perspirants? My doctor does not talk to me about deodorant and anti-perspirants. It is not good for anyone to wear an anti-perspirant because that blocks you from sweating and you are supposed to sweat. When looking to buy a natural deodorant buy one without aluminum. It would not hurt to even buy an unscented deodorant. Do you need to wear deodorant all the time? Do you sweat a lot? Are you going to be exercising and sweating profusely today? Do you really need deodorant every day, are you even going to be leaving the house today? Just remember you are putting deodorant on your skin, near lymph nodes, and every chemical you put on your skin gets into your body and processed by your liver. Try to minimize the amount of perfumes, lotions, deodorant and other chemicals you put on your body. Give your liver a break whenever you can.

Chances are if something is good for you inside, it is good for you outside. If it is bad for you outside, chances are it is bad for you inside. If probiotics are good for me inside, they are good for me outside. Greek yogurt has probiotics and probiotics increase gut health. Greek yogurt, because of the probiotics, makes for a great facial cleanser. You can make a cheap, healthy facial scrub with plain Greek yogurt, honey and raw oatmeal. Another very healthy facial is to use plain Greek yogurt, honey and avocado. Has your doctor ever told you that probiotics are good for you inside and outside? If it is bad for you outside, it is bad for you inside. Remember using lotions, sprays, and chemicals on your skin soak into your body and is processed by your liver. It is not good to put all those chemicals on the outside of your body and cannot be good for inside your body.

I always wonder why people use shaving cream to shave their legs. You already are using soap and lathering up, do you really need to be using shaving cream? Again, think of the added chemicals you are putting on your skin that gets into your body. I know marketing states that we get a better, smoother, closer shave using shaving cream, but really doesn't soap do the same thing? Has your doctor ever talked to you about shaving cream? I did not think so that is why I am telling you.

The doctor is not going to ask if you are constipated, have diarrhea, or ask if your stools are normal like a cigar. Okay, the doctor may ask these questions, but he is not going to change your diet based on your answer. Your doctor may prescribe medicine to stop whatever symptom you are currently having. As a Certified Health Coach, first I am going to ask what you are eating or drinking that may be causing these symptoms. It is normal to have at least one bowel movement a day and two bowel movements a day is good too. If you are not eliminating daily, it definitely could be your diet and you should seriously change your food intake so you will be having a bowel movement at least daily. It is amazing to me that a banana that is green can help stop diarrhea and a really ripe banana will help with constipation. The same fruit can have two different effects depending on the ripeness of the banana, I find that truly amazing. Does your doctor tell you that a green banana has less sugar than a really ripe banana? Think about that, really ripe bananas are used to make sweet breads, like banana bread.

Does your doctor ask you if you are practicing mindful eating? Mindful eating means that you are actually present, in the moment, when you eat, you are aware of what you are eating, not being stressed or rushed when you eat. Mindful eating means you are sitting to eat your food and not sitting in a car and driving while eating. Mindful eating is seeing your food, actually tasting your food, smelling your food, chewing slowly, just being in the moment and slowing down to enjoy your food. Have you ever eaten when you were angry or stressed and ate so fast that you cannot even remember eating? Have you ever overeaten because you were driving while you ate or you were eating while sitting in front of the television or computer? These are not practices of someone who is implementing mindful eating. When you chew your food, ensure you are chewing each bite at least 20 to 30 times. This helps break down your food and helps to start the digestion of your food so the rest of your digestive system does not have to work so hard. I know sometimes I hold on to my fork and I am already putting more food in my mouth to chew even before I chewed and swallowed the current bite of food. Have you ever done that? Lately, I think to myself, "what are you doing picking up your fork, put down your fork, you have not even chewed this bite 20 times, put down your fork and chew your food?" Just thinking that to myself is helping me to slow down and count how many times I am actually chewing each bite of food. Repeating that statement to myself after each bite takes at least 10 seconds and helps me to ensure I am chewing my food longer and eating slower. Practice mindful eating each and every time you put any food in your mouth.

Taking time to say a prayer to bless your food before you eat is another great way to practice mindful eating. Just the prayer itself to bless your food helps you to slow down, be in the moment and just calms you down so you do not eat so fast.

Exercise does help you to have overall better health. If you are ever given the choice, to eat healthy or to exercise, choose to eat healthy. Eating healthy is better for you than exercise and it is a lot simpler to eat healthy than to exercise. I do not know about you, but after I eat healthy I do not need to go take a shower as I do after I exercise. Remember you cannot exercise your way out of a poor diet. Eating healthy and exercise do go hand-in-hand but it is better for you to eat healthy than to exercise. It is easier to start with cleaning up the foods you eat and then later add in exercise. If you are eating healthy the weight will come off naturally. If you are able, you could start to exercise the same time you begin eating healthy.   Most people like to lose some weight first, feel better and have more energy and then start an exercise program while they are continuing to eat healthy.

I went to the gym the other day basically to use the sauna to sweat out my toxins. While I was in the sauna I just casually started asking how long everyone has been coming to this gym. One lady said that she works out 2 to 4 hours a day for years and cannot seem to lose weight. I asked her if she thought her diet had anything to do with that. She said she never used to eat breakfast and now she has one hard-boiled egg every morning. First of all, that is not eating breakfast because it is not a well-balanced meal, not enough calories, vitamins, protein, and not enough to hold her over until her snack or her next meal. She never even thought that her diet had anything to do with her having to feel the need to work out 2 to 4 hours a day for years without being able to lose weight.   Eating healthy has everything to do with being healthy. You cannot exercise your way out of a poor diet! I felt sorry for her because she feels the need to work out that many hours a day, she is not seeing results with her weight coming down and that she has not even thought to change her diet. I felt sorry for her because she has not yet learned what I learned a few years ago, that it is more important to eat healthy than to exercise so hard. It is simple to eat healthy and more difficult to work out because you need the time and equipment to work out. She is where I was for so many years, thinking I could eat anything I wanted, basically eat poorly, and expecting to exercise the poor food choices off. However, if she was eating healthy, her weight would be coming off naturally. If she continued to exercise, her weight would come off even more with the combination of eating healthy and exercise. She has chosen to exercise several hours a day instead of trying to look at her diet and eat healthier, that however is not the path I would recommend you all take. I am strongly encouraging you to always look at your diet, the foods you eat, first and foremost before you try anything else. Change what you can and that is always your diet. Always start with the foods you are eating or not eating as the beginning to improving your health.

Many years ago, when I was in the military, I did go see a nutritionist. To my surprise, she told me that pasta should never be a main dish but always a side dish. So now I am sharing that with you, pasta should never be a main dish but always a side dish. Has your doctor told you not to eat pasta as a main dish but to eat it as a side dish? I did not think so that is why I am telling you. It is better to have a serving of pasta, a vegetable and a protein with it and not just a large plate of pasta. Eating pasta as a main dish is a lot of complex carbohydrates to be eating and digesting. After eating a lot of carbohydrates like that, or white rice or pizza, you are going to be tired. To make pasta healthier, you can start eating it as a side dish and not a main dish. Eating brown rice pasta, black bean pasta, sprouted grain pasta are all better options for you than to eat plain white pasta or white rice. Zucchini sliced thin as a noodle is better for you than spaghetti because it has less carbohydrates and it is a vegetable so it is healthier for you. Be aware of the sauces you choose to put on your pasta. Most pasta sauces have a lot of sugar and sodium. Both sugar and salt are flavor enhancers and will cause you to eat more than a serving size of sauce. You could use extra virgin olive oil, diced fresh tomatoes and herbs instead of a store-bought pasta sauce. Making your own healthier sauce is always an option too then you can control the ingredients in the sauce. You could even add in things like garlic, onions, chopped carrots, diced tomatoes, green peppers, basically whatever you like and want in your sauce other than sugar and salt.

Eat an apple before you go to the grocery store. Has your doctor ever told you to eat an apply before you go grocery shopping? Probably your doctor has not even discussed this with you, so again, I will. When you have an apple before you go shopping, you will not be hungry as you shop. When you are not hungry as you are shopping, you will more likely stick to your grocery list because you will not be grabbing things just because you are hungry. When you eat an apple before you shop, you are more likely to buy healthier foods when you shop because you ate a healthy snack before you shopped. I do not know about you, but I am going to eat an apple before I go to the store if it helps me to shop for healthier foods.

Watch the size of your smoothies. It is so easy to put a lot of ingredients into the blender and the next thing you know you just made a smoothie that should be for 2 or 3 people. But you end up drinking it all by yourself in one smoothie. It is okay to drink part of the smoothie when it is made and drink part later as a snack or as your next meal. When I make smoothies, they are not always for taste but for nutritious value. I like to use the guidelines of three vegetables to one fruit when making smoothies.

You do not need to be eating meat at every meal. Has your doctor talked to you about not eating so much meat? If you eat meat, eating meat 1 to 2 times a week is plenty of times to be eating meat. You can get your protein from other food sources like beans, nuts, and if you eat dairy then cottage cheese and yogurt are other sources of protein. When buying meat, ensure you are buying farm raised, free roaming, hormone free, and basically the best meats you can buy. How much protein a person needs is up to each individual person to learn how much and what type of protein is best for them to be consuming. Some people do better on different types of protein. Maybe you would do well with protein powder instead of meat all the time. Try different proteins to see if the proteins hold you over or not. If you want to use protein powders, then I recommend trying different protein powders, different brands and different flavors to see which ones you like.

Does your doctor talk to you about portion size or about getting back to the basics? Meaning it is okay and recommended to order the small or regular size and not the large or jumbo size. Think "getting back to the basics" as what size was around when you were growing up. Places did not offer super-size back then so why do you need to order it now? Growing up the dinner plates were 8 inches and now dinner plates are 12 inches. Have you thought about going back to an 8-inch plate to eat your meals? If you are eating healthy all the time or most of the time, then a 12-inch plate does not matter because you will fill it with mostly vegetables. If you are eating poorly you may want to use a smaller size plate until you are eating healthier so you get used to seeing normal portion sized foods.

Just because something is sold in a health food store, that does not mean it is healthy for you. I have never had a doctor mention al health food store to me, have you? Again, think about your goal, what is your goal? There are many different protein powders in a health food store so if you are cutting out dairy than you will not want to purchase a protein powder with whey. All those granola bars or drinks are not always healthy and have way more than 5 ingredients. If your goal is to be eating less processed foods, than maybe you may not want to shop in a health food store for lots of items. Do not misunderstand me, I am not against health food stores. There are a lot of good things in a health food store, just be wise and know your goal when you walk in.

Just because you are purchasing processed organic food, it still may contain more than 5 ingredients even though all ingredients are organic. If eating less than 5 ingredients is one of your goals, you must read labels, even on organic foods. I am always trying to cut out added sugars. Even organic processed foods may have added organic sugar.

In my house, we say "some is better than none." We may not always want to eat the entire carrot or a whole avocado so eating some is better than eating none. You will still get the benefits of the vegetable or fruit without eating the entire vegetable or fruit. "Some is better than none" is a great concept for smoothies, salads, or when having a plate of vegetables as a snack. You may not like a certain vegetable so eating some may get your palate to start liking that vegetable. Anytime you are trying a new fruit, vegetable or anything like Kiefer, remember some is better than none. Has your doctor ever talked to you about eating some is better than none?

Also in my house, we say "something is better than nothing." It is better to do 5 minutes of exercise or cleaning than to do nothing at all. It is better to do anything rather than to sit and do nothing. It is better to work in your closet putting clothes away for 5 minutes than to let your closet get piled up of clothing. A little bit is better than nothing. Of course, the more you do the more chances you have to make mistakes. It is easy to sit on the couch all day and do nothing. Something is better than nothing, just get up and be moving. Remember, if you always do what you have always done you will always get the same results. We want different results this time, right?

Doctors may not tell you how you should not be drinking all those meal replacements, taking all those weight loss pills, mixing those chemicals into your drinks but I am telling you not to do it. Think of all those chemicals you are putting into your body. Try to find healthier ways to be getting those ingredients, in their natural state, instead of in a drink, shake, stick or whatever it may be called on your plan. Are you going to be eating or rather "drinking" this way for life? Probably not because it would get too costly and not be good on your body for life to be practicing this way of eating. You will still need to learn to eat healthy after you stop practicing this way of eating. It is so much easier to learn to eat healthy and do it for life than to be drinking weight loss drinks and putting chemicals into your body.

Has your doctor ever told you to rinse off your canned food, fresh fruits and vegetables? Rinse off canned food to get off some of the salt and preservatives, it cannot hurt. Rinse anything that you can rinse. Wash your fresh fruits and vegetables prior to eating them to get off preservatives and other germs from people touching the food in the store. Even if you are not going to eat the skin, rinse your fruits and vegetables because your knife goes through the skin into your fruit and vegetable and that is what you are going to be eating. Rinse your fruits and vegetables just before eating them so they will not get moldy or mushy from being rinsed and stored in the refrigerator.

With all this information on eating healthy, how are you going to implement all this new knowledge moving forward? I have a few ideas to help you as you continue moving forward.

Chapter 8

Moving Forward

Whatever you do, do not quit now! Quitting is not an option. You have come so far, learned so much, do no stop now on your eating healthy journey. It is a lifestyle to be eating healthy and not a diet. Continue to eat healthier every day. Continue on with what you have learned. If there are ideas in this book that you have not tried or implemented into your daily lifestyle, now is a good time to start with those ideas that you have not tried. Maybe as you were reading this book, ideas came to you that you would like to try or experiment with and now is a good time to try new things. Continue to make the healthiest possible food choices every day and everywhere you go. Remember, it really is simple to eat healthy.

As you move forward on your eating healthy journey, ask yourself if you need to change up your goals in any way. Maybe you have reached a goal by now and you will need to set new goals. Maybe you have realized that your goal changed and your original goal was not what you really wanted anyhow, so write new goals and stay focused on those new goals. Keep reevaluating your goals every few months to make sure you are staying the course to eating healthy.

Remember your eating healthy journey is exactly that, it is your journey. It is not a race to be won. It is not anyone else's pace but your pace. Continue to implement new healthier foods at a pace that is comfortable for you. Continue to try a new recipe maybe once a month, or once a week, whatever is comfortable for you.

Look for ways that you can add in one healthy meal. Maybe it is to go meatless one meal a week. Maybe you can add in more vegetables into your meals. Begin eating vegetables as a snack instead of eating junk for a snack. Look for ways to make your meals healthier by continuing to make healthier food swaps. Keep telling yourself "I know there is a way that I can make this meal healthier" and figure out what that would be for you for each meal.

Forming new habits will take time. It took time to develop your old bad habits and it will take time to form your new good eating habits. For every bad, negative eating habit that you are trying to replace with a new, healthy eating habit, be patient and it will develop into a new habit. It may just happen overnight for you that you switch to eating healthier foods, and that would be awesome but it if does not happen overnight, continue to make your new eating habit a routine. We all like routines and eating healthier is no different. Get in a good daily routine of eating healthy and it will get simpler as time goes along.

Make a difference in the world by spreading information on eating healthy. Get involved in groups that are health conscious, with like-minded people and share ideas how you can spread health information to others. Maybe start small and prepare a healthy dish or meal and invite in one neighbor to talk to them about eating healthier. Maybe have a neighborhood picnic and ask everyone to bring a healthy dish to share.

Swap healthy recipes with your family and friends to build your healthy recipe collection. Look for ways to make your favorite recipes even healthier.

Start reading healthy, clean eating magazines. Try a new recipe each month or each week out of your healthy eating magazines.

Be the one that your family, friends, and co-workers see ordering a healthy meal when you eat out. Discuss with them that you are making your health a priority and you are choosing healthier foods and healthier meals to eat. Be the one in restaurants to ask for a side of two steamed vegetables instead of getting the sides that normally come with the meal. Let others see you eating the healthy foods. Set the example for your family, friends and co-workers to follow.

Be an encourager. Encourage others to join you and come along side you on your healthy journey. When you see someone walking in the neighborhood or eating a healthy meal, talk to them, congratulate them on getting out there and becoming healthier. Encouraging someone just may be the extra push of motivation that they need to stick with it. Ask others to go for a walk with you. Start a neighborhood walking group or exercise group.

Be creative. If you do not have junk food in your house, you will have to be creative when a snack attack comes along. It is fun! Try different combinations of foods to get that desire you are craving. If you want something sweet, maybe have a green tea or herbal tea with a little honey to curb your sweet tooth. Maybe eat a ripe banana with raw almond butter and a tad of honey. Moving forward, do not bring junk foods in the house. Eat fruit or a sweet vegetable when you want something sweet.

Write letters to grocery stores or restaurants and let them know what they are doing that is healthy that you like. Maybe they are offering more organic foods. Maybe they are offering more healthy choices on the menu. Or write the grocery stores or restaurants and let them know you would like to see more healthy foods being carried in the store and more vegetarian meals on the menu.

If you help the homeless or shelters by preparing meals or delivering meals to those places, start to prepare healthier foods. The people in shelters deserve to eat healthier too. Do not always take them foods like pizza, fried chicken or donuts but start dropping off fruit and fruit trays or salad bar type foods.

Another thing I would like to see in the world moving forward with the ripple effect of good health is that instead of saying "I lost weight" or "I dropped so many pounds" we start to say something more positive. Subconsciously, when we "lose" something, we want to find it. When we "drop" something, we want to pick it up. Why do we say "I lost weight" and now that makes us want to find it? Why do we say "I dropped so many pounds"? Then we want to pick up what we "dropped." Let's start saying things like "Eat Healthy to Be Healthy." Or say things like "I'm eating healthier." Let's start focusing on how eating healthier makes us feel instead of focusing on the number we see on the scale.

CONCLUSION

Thank you everyone for allowing me the opportunity to come alongside of you on your eating healthy journey. It has been a real pleasure for me and I hope for you as well. Remember: *"Eat Healthy, Be Healthy - It Is That Simple!"* Starting anything is always the hardest part, and starting to eat healthy is no exception. I wanted to give you many simple ideas to get you started to eat healthy. There is more to eating healthy than I wrote about here in this book, but I wanted to just get you to start eating better. By now you have started eating healthier and you are well on your way to eating healthier. We make eating healthy more complicated than it has to be. It is simple to eat healthy. Make yourself and your health a priority, eat healthy for you. Do at least one thing a day toward your goal of eating healthier to be healthier. Keep eating healthy as simple as possible, then you will do it for life. I would like to leave you with this thought "no turning back," continue on your healthy eating journey!

This book was inspired by my experience at the Institute for Integrative Nutrition® (IIN), where I received my training in holistic wellness and health coaching.

IIN offers a truly comprehensive Health Coach Training Program that invites students to deeply explore the things that are most nourishing to them. From the physical aspects of nutrition and eating wholesome foods that work best for each individual person, to the concept of Primary Food – the idea that everything in life, including our spirituality, career, relationships, and fitness contributes to our inner and outer health – IIN helped me reach optimal health and balance. This inner journey unleashed the passion that compels me to share what I have learned and inspire others.

Beyond personal health, IIN offers training in health coaching, as well as business and marketing. Students who choose to pursue this field professionally complete the program equipped with the communication skills and branding knowledge they need to create a fulfilling career encouraging and supporting others in reaching their own health goals.

From renowned wellness experts as Visiting Teachers to the convenience of their online learning platform, this school has changed my life, and I believe it will do the same for you. I invite you to learn more about the Institute for Integrative Nutrition and explore how the Health Coach Training Program can help you transform your life.

Feel free to contact me to hear more about my personal experience at lizgraybill@yahoo.com, or call (844) 315-8546 to learn more.

About the Author

Liz Graybill served her country in the U.S. Army and retired after 23 years of Honorable service. While in the Army, she was overweight for the last 18 years of her military career. She was overweight, tired all the time, had no energy, then diagnosed with hypothyroidism (underactive thyroid). After retiring from the Army, her weight kept increasing and she hit her all time highest weight. She then started her journey of eating healthy, lost 30 pounds, and has kept the weight off. She gained energy and went off medication for hypothyroidism. While on her journey to eat healthy, she became a Certified Health Coach. As a Certified Health Coach, she now helps people to eat healthy, lose weight, and hold them accountable to reach their goals of being healthy.

Liz and her husband Doug are the Founders of a non-profit, Veterans Making A Difference. They help veterans in need in Berks County, Pennsylvania. Being called into something more for veterans, they recently opened the Paul R Gordon Veteran Social Center in Reading, Pennsylvania, where they will be able to help more veterans.

Invite Liz to Speak to
Your Group or Organization

Liz is a very passionate speaker on the topics of nutrition, healthy eating, healthier food swaps, losing weight, sleep and anything related to eating healthy.

Liz brings a lot of enthusiasm and knowledge on making healthier choices and doing so for life not as a diet.

Liz has spoken to several audiences including:

- Glad Tidings Church Loving Arms Group for emotional and spiritual needs for cancer patients

- Senior Berners Group on Healthy Eating

- Utilities Employees Credit Union during Lunch and Learn on Sleep

- Has also lead many small groups on healthy eating as a lifestyle and leads the monthly Meatless Monday small group at her church.